Don't Look Ba

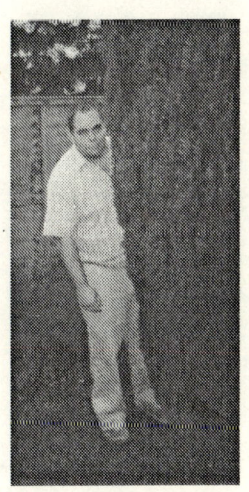

By Phillip Pettican

All rights reserved, no part of this publication may be reproduced by any means, electronic, mechanical, or photocopying. No documentary or film without prior permission of the publisher.

Published by
Chipmunkapublishing
PO Box 6872
Brentwood
Essex Cm13 1ZT
United Kingdom

Copyright © 2003 Chipmunkapublishing

A record of this book is in the British Library
ISBN **0954221869**

Printed and bound
In Great Britain.

As Chipmunka's author list grows, it shows that mental distress affects everyone, from all walks of life. Chipmunkapublishing is unique in that it allows ordinary people to tell their extraordinary stories.

Phil's story is touching and poignant. He was an ordinary guy, serving in the Navy and working as a builder, before mental distress turned his world upside down.

He writes his story with an empathic simplicity that you can't help but feel the terrible isolation that is mental illness. He tries to be an ordinary guy again, but as anyone who has gone through similar experiences knows, it changes, for better or for worse, your life forever.

There is no happily ever after in this book, the soul triumphs, but there is still the washing up to do… and more pain to face. Believing in reincarnation, he hopes for a better life next time around. Phil, I hope this book will make this one a little better. You deserve it.
A good autobiography is when you not only know and understand the person writing, but love them too.

Dolly Sen Author and Mental Health Activist

THE SHAPE OF THINGS TO COME

From an early stage in my life there were signs that things were slightly amiss.

As a baby I used to cry a lot especially when I was put to bed, as soon as I was left alone for the night I would start. According to my mother they tried everything to stop me crying but without success. So in the end I was left to get on with it. Apparently this went on for several months. Thinking back I can vaguely remember the feelings of terrible loneliness and isolation felt at this period in time.

As I grew up I became aware of how little us children saw of our father, this however to little children was accepted as normal, probably because we knew nothing different. On the occasions we did see him it was very exciting to us because it was such a rare event and he sometimes brought 'things' home. It was nice to see Dad, why couldn't we see him more often?
As you may have gathered I had a big sister called Susan (Sue) although there is only 2 years between us, it seemed a huge gap especially when she started school and left me on my own! I was still very young and I had lost my main playmate, at least in the daytime. I seem to remember that this was the first period in my life when I had to come to terms with being alone.

Adjustment came and so there I was playing with my toys and inventing little games with them (this may seem a normal occurrence, especially for a little boy of 3 or 4 years of age), games which would develop and expand as I became older.

As I approached school age I began to know more

of the other children on the housing estate where I lived, mainly due to Susan befriending them at school. Susan was still my main friend and I used to look forward to her coming home every day so we could go out and play. However, during school days I became used to spending hours on my own. I must hasten to add that Mum did not neglect us children and I often went out to the shops and other places with her! But gradually I came to enjoy playing by myself and used to spend hours in a red pedal car which I had. Little did I know that in the future I would have to spend a lot more time amusing myself!

Time marched on and the dreaded day of going to school came along. So there I was walking hand in hand with Mum in my posh uniform approaching those enormous gates and the massive school buildings, with its large classroom and all those strange little faces and the big beaming smile of the lady teacher. After the initial introductions Mum said her goodbyes and disappeared out of the door, leaving me there with all those gawping little faces. It was too much, up I jumped, flung the door open, and ran in hot pursuit of that cruel, heartless lady who had left me in that awful place. I ran and ran until Mum was in sight, then on seeing her burst into tears and begged her not to take me there again. She did!

The school in question was King's Road County Junior in Chelmsford, Essex and I was to spend what seemed all my days there until I reached the age of 11. As schools go it was not bad and it was there I learnt to read and write. The headmaster was certainly a character or should I say fearful character. He was a Welshman with a typical Welshman's voice. Catch him in a bad mood and then watch out. He used to go on the warpath, parading up and down the school corridors, cane in hand, shouting threats at the poor pupils who were passing his way. As I became older and got to know him through various means, he started to earn my respect and by the time I left that school I liked him.

My early childhood was fairly normal, going to school and coming home to Mum and Susan. During this time I learnt to ride a bike and consequently spent a lot of my spare time riding it.

When weekends came along we used to see Dad. If we were lucky enough he used to take us into Chelmsford on Saturdays. I never really worked out where he went all the time because he used to leave us in the car for long periods of time. When Susan was doing other things I went with him alone. After doing the necessary errands on the Saturdays more often than not he would park somewhere and tell me he would not be long and then disappear for up to 2 hours. Thinking back I used to get very bored and tried to practice my imaginary driving skills, sometimes leaving the car in gear. Of course, on returning, Dad would start the car and it would jolt forward. Then came the reprimand!

I was seven years of age when my life changed. It was what seemed a normal Saturday. Dad and I went into the city, did a few things and then went to a place I'd never been before. We parked adjacent to a large building. Expecting to be left alone again I was most surprised when Dad told me to come with him. We entered the building and went into a lift which began to take us upwards, nearly to the top. Soon we were standing outside a door at which Dad produced a key and proceeded to open it. It was a flat. I did not understand why we were there but found it quite exciting, it was certainly different from where we had been living! Dad showed me around and then told me

that this was where he would be living. I did not understand. Why would he be living there and not all of us? It still had not sunk in when we arrived home. I decided to find Mum and Susan, and tell them. Meanwhile Dad had gone!
Mum explained that Dad had decided to leave us and would not be coming back and that the flat was indeed where he was going to live. It took a while for me to come to terms with what Mum had said. I did not understand why Dad would leave us, what I did know was that I was devastated. All three of us were upstairs in Mum and Dad's bedroom crying our eyes out.
Things never seemed the same after that fateful day and I, for one, never thought I would ever recover from it.

Life goes on, and so it did, but differently. Mum was different; she was not as tolerant as she had been. We did not understand!
    Dad came to see us, of course, mainly at weekends. He usually took us to that flat and not only to that flat, but to that nasty woman as well! Yes, he had a friend, a woman friend and she was horrible! Everything I did and said was wrong. She made my life a misery! Initially after all the turmoil had calmed down, Susan and I started staying at the flat, normally on a Saturday night. This, however, did not last long as Hazel (Dad's friend) continued behaving badly. Every night I stayed, whilst I was trying to sleep in the bedroom all I could hear was Dad and Hazel arguing about me, always me and my so called bad behaviour and bad manners. The arguments were always heated, and looking back, always trivial - even about the way I held my knife and fork at meal times. Soon the arguments became threats. Threats of intent to come into my bedroom and inflict discipline,

either verbal or physical and I was terrified. I could hear every word that was said and it went on sometimes for an hour or more! I would lay there shaking, every time I heard that voice going on and on. I was petrified. What was happening to me? What was happening in my life? Why did Dad live with that person, that witch?
I stopped going to Dad's flat, it was all too much. I did not like her and I told him so. He said I should not be so silly and come and see him. But I was adamant that even if it meant seeing less of Dad I would not go again.

Of course, I told Mum all about it and she was sympathetic. Susan still went to see Dad as Hazel did not seem to bother her. Why didn't she like me? I had never been naughty to her, why didn't she leave me alone? I was upset, and baffled by the injustice of it all.
School days continued regardless, and I indulged in various sporting activities and became involved with the school choir. Football was my first love and I played in the school team. Playing football helped me forget my troubles at home, but I began to notice that my playing ability used to fluctuate. One day I would be relaxed and confident and therefore reflect it in my playing, the next I would be tense and ill at ease and consequently play terribly. This acted to reinforce my already dwindling self-confidence. This fluctuating form, in sport in general was unknowingly at the time going to frustrate me throughout my life.

It was about this time that I found out that the school had a famous former pupil. His name was Geoff Hurst and played football for West Ham. The headmaster noticed the interest in Mr Hurst and arranged a visit to go and watch him play and also to meet the man and his team as well.

So, one Saturday, a coach load of excited children

arrived at the football ground to watch West Ham play Sheffield United. We were able to watch the match from a viewing box in the main grandstand. We felt very important and all of us were given mementos and souvenirs of the visit. Our headmaster even tried to arrange for us to go into the changing room to meet the players, but unfortunately was unsuccessful. So we had to be content with waiting outside the player's entrance to catch a glimpse of our heroes. We waited and waited but they never emerged, so we had to leave without meeting them, it was so disappointing!

One thing that did develop personally from the visit was my love affair with West Ham United, which continues to this day.

My other talent which didn't change with the weather was singing. I had an excellent singing voice and it was not long before I was called on to do solos at school concerts and so on. Through this I developed a small celebrity status among other pupils and teachers which I enjoyed, especially as I was now one of the older children!

However, I was not alone with my gift, I had a rival! His name was Francis Moore and was in the Chelmsford Cathedral Choir. He had more confidence than me and came from a well off family, he considered himself best.

Unfortunately I also considered him better than me but this only served to make me more resilient in not showing my feelings of inferiority. Our rivalry grew. I joined my local church choir after turning down an audition for the Cathedral - I made sure that Francis knew this. We were then entered into various singing recitals and even competitions.

Our rivalry came to a head in the playground one

day when we started pushing each other around. The headmaster heard about our scuffle and decided a proper boxing match would be in order. So a day was arranged and we were both issued with boxing gloves.

The battle commenced with many interested spectators and the headmaster as referee. This was really the first fight I had ever had and at first I was reluctant to hit my opponent, whereas he had no reluctance at all. I was knocked all over the place! When I did manage to hit back I surprised myself and found an aggressiveness I never realised I had. Francis won the boxing match but I felt good that I could indeed fight back.

As my days at King's Road were coming to an end I grew to like the headmaster. He was also a singer and often encouraged me in my exploits and was also sympathetic about my parents split. He had my respect and affection and I missed him when I left.
Looking back, my early school days were my happiest.

About a year before Dad left my Grandad died. I didn't know him that well so his death did not affect me much. It affected Mum because he was her father!

What did affect me was the fact that we moved house. We moved into Nana's house and little did I know how much it would affect me. Nanna was an old lady and she was crippled with arthritis and used to get around on sticks which doubled as weapons!

Things were not too bad at first, but after a while my home life deteriorated once again. Mum was forced to go out to work and she worked in the evenings which left Susan and I at home with Nanna.

Now Nanna had her own room which was the next room to our sitting room, so any noise or misbehaviour could be heard easily. Susan and I were now of an age where we began to fight each other both verbally and physically.

I tried to be good for Mum's sake but Susan used to bait me because she knew that Nanna always thought it was my fault and therefore passed that information on. Every night when Mum came home she would hear the news that 'that boy' had been naughty again.

It all became too much for Mum one night and when she came home and received the usual report, she snapped, came upstairs, stormed into my bedroom and woke me up by smacking me. At this stage I realised things were getting out of control and I had been unjustly punished, so I spoke to Mum and told her it was not always me who misbehaved and that Nanna blamed me for everything!

After that things started to improve a little, Mum mellowed towards me and began to believe that it was not all my fault. Susan stopped trying to bait me but very soon we began to antagonise Nanna. We used to pretend to misbehave so Nanna would come into the room and wave her sticks at me, and then we would laugh at her. Nanna would try and hit me with her sticks but was never able to hurt me, but I pretended she did.

Apart from being the end of the week Fridays became special for me. Every Friday night we saw Dad, he used to take us to see Granny and Granddad (his father and mother). Sometimes he would bring presents I liked. I enjoyed seeing Dad and I liked going to Witham. Granny and Granddad were so nice to me and sometimes I even stayed with them.

They went to church on Sundays and when I stayed I went with them. Religion was encouraged by Mum, and Susan and I used to go to Sunday school which I didn't like. One Sunday on the way to the

Methodist Church which we attended, I suddenly panicked and decided I could not face it. So I left Susan and turned round and walked back home. I was so frightened that Mum would be angry with me, that by the time I reached home I was crying. But Mum wasn't angry and never made me go again.

One day a strange man came to see us or rather came round with Mum. He was bald and spoke with a Scottish accent. We were to see a lot more of him and it was not long before we were going out with him in his big car. We even went round to his flat some Sundays for dinner which I remember well because he used to carry Nanna up the stairs, I thought he was very strong. We called him Uncle Tom.

Uncle Tom became part of our lives, and it soon became apparent that my life was about to change yet again. By this time I was getting used to upheaval and learned to accept different situations. I adjusted the best I could and was reaching the age where I was beginning to understand them. I had lived my first decade. However, in hindsight, despite initial understanding I was still feeling insecure, past experiences had left their scars.

I was now in the Cub Scouts and again, like school, I was always initially reluctant to attend. As soon as I arrived and got involved in the activities I even enjoyed it.

One weekend I went camping with all the other boys, it was not very far from home but it was the first time I had ever been away. We set up camp and were settling in when I experienced my first pangs of home sickness. I didn't understand the feelings of terrible isolation and loneliness and was very relieved when

Mum and Uncle Tom came to visit me that evening. I told them how I felt and said that I wanted to go home. They said I could if I wanted to but that these horrible feelings would disappear. I was persuaded to stay and enjoyed the rest of the weekend.

Having reached the age of 11, I took the 11 plus examination and passed and now all I was waiting for was to find out my new school. I was waiting with trepidation; it would mean another upheaval in my life, leaving the school I had been at for years and everything familiar that goes with it.

Up until then every traumatic experience that had happened to me had occurred in my home surroundings and not at school. So I always had a steadying influence to fall back on, but now even that had gone! There was more to come.

We were moving again. Not just in Chelmsford but far, far away to a place called Hethersett, near Norwich.

GROWING UP

We moved to a village called Hethersett, near Norwich. Mum and Uncle Tom were in love and decided to live together, so Susan and I and Tom's children - Kenneth and Alistair - went with them.

It was a brand new house on a new housing estate, and it was all very strange and intimidating to me. So many new things at once to get accustomed to: new house; new village; new school and Uncle Tom's sons who were a couple of years younger than me. They were twins, although they didn't look it. Alastair was at least 6 inches taller than Kenneth who was really quite small for his age.

The first thing to cope with was school. My new school was a daily bus ride away; it was called Wymondham College and was an unusual place with most of the classrooms being Nissen huts. It was both a boarding school and a day school, and to begin with the two were kept apart.

I settled in slowly, initially I had to deal with the other children taking the mickey out of my Essex accent. Instead of ignoring the jibes I tended to let it upset me and, of course, provoked more criticism. Eventually I was accepted and soon after learning to cope with the mental bullying it stopped.

My first year through school in Norfolk passed without incident. My workload, especially homework, was a new burden to contend with and I coped the best I could. I found there were always a distraction both at

home and school that used to affect my concentration, this was to continue for the rest of my school days.
Home life after the move took longer to settle down. The school being miles away meant most school friends lived around Norwich. I was never one to have many friends throughout my life; I preferred to have relationships with the odd one or two people.

The house was big and had four bedrooms so I was lucky to have my own room, with Susan in one and the twins in the other. Relationships tended to fluctuate, with the twins tending to stick together, especially when things became hot. Uncle Tom was strict and was not averse to smacking, so I soon learned how not to upset him, although of course with four children in the house that was not always easy.

Nanna was still living with us but was affected by deteriorating health. She had her bed in the dining room and tended to spend most of the time in there.
Mum had her hands full with so many mouths to feed, and clothes to wash and, of course, house to clean. She was happier now but sometimes things still got on top of her and she had to let off steam now and again.

During the early months I formed a friendship with the two boys from over the road. They did not attend my school so I saw them mainly at weekends. It was not a close friendship but it was nice to associate with boys of my own age when away from school.

I was out one day with one of them when we met up with a couple of the local tough boys, whose names were Sammy Knot and Jason Roberts. Sammy and Jason were friendly enough at first but I did not trust them, and sure enough it was not long before they started having fun at our expense. They cornered us in a cul-de-sac not far from home and it was obvious they were not going let us through without a fight. After deliberation we decided to try our luck and dash through them, which we did. I made it, but my mate was not so lucky and was beaten up! By the time I returned to the scene of the crime everyone had gone. I met up with my mate later - he was not too badly hurt, but our relationship was. I could not understand why he was so upset; if I had gone back I would have been beaten up as well! One thing I did know is that I was frightened and the thought never crossed my mind to go back. Reputations can be true or false. Sammy Knot and Jason Roberts had reputations and I was to meet them again.

My first year in Ethernet was very insignificant and mundane, both my school and home life were to take a complete change in direction.

It was 1969 and I was 12 years old. September was the end of the holiday and back to school. Everybody had been graded since the first year and therefore put in different classes; consequently new faces appeared in my life yet again.

There was one new face that interested me more than the others, he had been on the bus that brought us to school and also lived in Ethernet - a potential friend perhaps! Sure enough it was not long before we became friendly. His name was David Ward and had just moved from Kent, he lived just down the road from me in a newly built housing estate. Being in the same class we soon started to sit together in lessons and come the evenings, he used to call round to my house where I was allowed 'out to play' for a couple of hours.

David had a tougher background than I and soon started to dominate the relationship. He taught me various things, like acting tough and rebellious and it wasn't long before we experimented in smoking and spitting and other disgusting habits. For me it was only a temporary phase. I soon decided this new image was not for me, especially as I had been brought up to be good mannered and respectful and had to behave that way at home. However, David and I remained good mates and continued to get up to mischief both at home and at school!

Another new arrival at school was a face that I had come across before. He too used the same bus as David and I but was just starting his first term in a class a year below me. It was Jason Roberts, one half of the terrible duo I had met previously. The other half - Sammy Knot attended the local Secondary School being not as bright! Jason, David and I became mates and consequently after school used to meet up with Sammy. So there we were new friends and soon new reputations.

Jason and Sammy regarded David as their equal but with me it was different, I had things to prove. Friendly confrontation developed firstly at school with Jason and later at home with Sammy. Both of them often practiced fighting one another, this took the form of friendly wrestling matches and it was not long before I was drawn into them. Jason and I used to wrestle a lot on the school playing field and I found that I could more than hold my own. Of course, this was all well and good in friendly fights but if anything got out of hand and serious, trepidation would return.

However, Jason's reputation started to rub off on me and my association with David all helped to enhance my position. I was soon considered by other pupils to be someone to respect. It was a good feeling and one I quickly became accustomed to. I was not one to flaunt my toughness as that would create confrontation and besides I knew deep down I was and always will be just a big pussy-cat.

Occasionally I would encounter situations that required bluff to master my adversary, and found this was enough. Sometimes, very occasionally, a fight would ensue but these were few and far between. Some of these I will detail later.

The months were passing and my friendship with both David and Sammy was growing. Jason was history, he moved to Australia and wrote to Sammy for a while but the letters became few and far between.

I did not have the same reputation at home as at school, I did not want it! There were a lot of mean and hard children in Ethernet, most of them attended Sammy's school and I was out of their league. I was witness to some very brutal fights, some concerning Sammy. He was a very hard and tough boy, but was also a mate and I felt safe when I was with him.

I remember one day, a few local friends along with Sammy, David and I went blackcurrant picking. It was hard work but fun and there were lots of other boys doing the same. Two particular boys - not known by us - were taking the full brunt of our jokes and Mickey taking. I must add as usual I was not directly involved, only laughing at the fun. Most of our lot, including Sammy, went to get their pickings weighed leaving me with the two strangers in the next line. One of the boys came over to me and said his friend was not scared of me and was going to 'smash my face in'. Fear engulfed me yet again and I had no reply to the threats except to tell Sammy on his return. Without hesitation he went over to the boy, Hit him twice - once in the stomach and once in the face, and then calmly muttered to me that it was time to go home. It was so clinical!

I had reached puberty, my voice had broken and I was growing up. Nanna had a stroke and was deteriorating fast. Mum had her hands full at this time, what with four children and an invalid to look after as well as Uncle Tom. She coped well and even stopped trying to smack me - I was getting too big, and it did not hurt anymore! It was about this time that Mum started to become my friend and I started to confide in her a lot more.
Sue, my sister, had reached the awkward age and was becoming a rebel. She had a boyfriend and tended to spend all her time with him, often staying out later that she should, and when at home played the 'Rolling Stones' at full volume. There were many heated rows between (Uncle) Tom and her and they were never resolved. Sue became more and more rebellious. All the family worried about my sister not least because of her boy friend, he was a local yob and appeared not to have any attributes whatsoever. We all waited for her to see the light, it took a while but eventually she matured and grew out of that boy and became part of the family again.

    Nanna died, it was a release from suffering. It did not affect me very much, we had never got on. Mum coped well and I was pleased that some of her workload had died along with my Grandmother.

    Sue and I did not see much of Dad at this time, his relationship with Hazel continued and was cemented with them marrying suddenly - I, of course, celebrated the news! They had also moved away from Chelmsford and ended up getting a house in Witham, quite near Grandma and Granddad. Dad was also going abroad a lot - something to do with his job which involved making training films for the armed forces, especially the Navy.

Mum and Tom married as well in 1970 and, of course, Sue and I attended the wedding. The twins by this time had moved to Scotland with their mother who had won custody of them in the court. Tom was clearly affected by their absence and appeared to be in one bad mood after another, so Sue and I tended to avoid speaking to him in fear of his wrath!

When not at school I was out most of the time. Along with Sammy and David I had an evening paper round which provided me with additional money that came in very handy, especially as I had started smoking. My relationship with Sammy grew and it was not long before we were spending most of our time together, he became my best friend. Unfortunately we tended to leave David out of things for a while, so he started to give me a hard time at school. He knew he could bully me and get away with it - or thought he could - until one day in the classroom he kept kicking my chair all through the lesson, this along with verbal badgering started to wind me up to such an extent that I lost my temper. After the exit of the teacher at the end of the lesson I attacked David with a ferocity that scared both David and I. I remember to this day the look of surprise on David's face as I laid into him. I stopped before I did him any real harm, but it stopped the bullying, at least for a while! Sammy and I continued to get up to mischief and he even went down to Essex with me for a weekend to see Dad. I never went to Dad's on my own because of Hazel, she still resented me!

The two of us mates went and did everything together; he was a good friend and never once bullied me - not like David. Occasionally we would have friendly fights on the playing field or in his house and sometimes I would out wrestle him. This was a turn up for the books as he was one of the toughest boys in the village, and in my opinion definitely tougher than David although this was never proved.

Our close friendship lasted about a year and during that time I realised that I would probably never have such a close friend again. Eventually it was David who came between us, he started to hang around with us more and more and even started calling round Sammy's by himself. This spelt the end of the unique relationship and led to me opting out altogether for a few weeks. I was hurt and I was jealous, and it took time to come to terms with.

By the time I resumed contact with Sammy and David the closeness had gone forever. It was not long after that, that Sammy moved out of the area and I never saw him again.

David and I inevitably started 'hanging around' together again, only this time he was less domineering and it was an easier relationship. We were not in each others classes at school by this time, so didn't get on each others nerves so much!

My interest in the opposite sex increased with the years and by the time I was 15 I was desperate for my first encounter. Many boys at school had girl friends and I began to feel left out. I had attempted to ask several girls, but my lack of guts always got in the way until most proposals were made through a third party. I found even if I received a positive sign of interest from a girl, I still turned to jelly at the thought of communication with her. Initially I would force myself into such a state that all efforts failed miserably! It was so frustrating!

However, there were the odd few girls at school who liked a bit of fun and one in particular comes to mind, her name was Jenny Whitelaw. Now many boys knew what Jenny would do but only a few would pursue her - I was one of the few!

Many times, after class, me and one or two mates would remain in the classroom along with an apparently non-cooperative Jenny. Then, when alone, after not too much struggling we would grope our way over a very well developed young body. This ritual continued for sometime, each time we would get bolder, but after a while Jenny got herself a boy friend and did not allow us near her anymore.

Life outside school continued, with David and I getting involved in various pursuits. The village had a football team which I played for a couple of times, but after a promising start my form became erratic and I lost my place. It seemed that the harder I tried the worse I became. It was all very worrying!

My other love was cycle speedway. This was a sport with similar rules to normal speedway, only using push-bikes. These bikes were specially adapted, with no brakes and only one gear and had thick tread tyres. There were sometimes two meetings a week in the summer and everyone who took part was very keen, so competition for places was very hot. I was very proud when I gained my first place in the team. At last I had found something I was consistently good at!

Sport at school consisted mainly of Rugby in the winter and cricket in the summer. I was fairly competent at Rugby, but began to find I suffered from heartburn quite a lot which when mixed with vigorous exercise did not go well together.

I had reached the fifth form - my last year - the year of 'O Level Examinations', the year I had to decide on a career. By this time the borders and day pupils were integrated and I found myself in a class of mostly intelligent borders. I became aware of how far I was slipping behind academically, and knew I had to study more if I was to succeed. But I hated studying and besides there were so many other distractions at home. History was a subject I could not master and in the final few months I had virtually given it up. I still attended the lessons however even though the teacher and fellow pupils knew I was a lost cause. When you are a lost cause you tend to be taken less seriously by your classmates. This I tended to tolerate and even went along with to a certain extent. There was one particular boy though who was taking things too far. The situation, I realised, had to be rectified otherwise I would lose all credibility. This boy had started sitting in my seat and was doing it openly, believing that I would not object for whatever reason best known to him.

The boy in question had been bullied in the early years at school and I had once felt sorry for him. But more recently he had learnt that standing up to the bully would almost certainly stop the bullying itself! This was the case but unfortunately he had developed a taste for fighting and had also developed ideas above his station. His reputation had certainly gone to his head and he was starting to get extremely obnoxious, so obnoxious in fact that he was disliked by many people and besides that, he was ugly with it.

So, with the usual trepidation, I waited for the next history lesson which I had decided was to be the time of our confrontation. He played into my hands by sitting in my seat. As I approached he gave me a toothy sneer and on my demand refused to vacate his position. I grabbed him, and pulled him by the collar off the seat, he struggled but before he could do anything I had him pinned over the desk.

Everyone was cheering and I even started to relax, I had taken him and for good measure punched him a couple of times in the torso, before being warned of the teachers' imminent arrival. He never sat in my seat again!

It was getting to the stage now that all I wanted to do was to leave school. I had more or less made up my mind what I was going to do with my life. I was going to join the Royal Navy either as an officer cadet or as a rating, which obviously depended on my exam results. Dad was thrilled that I had chosen this particular career and rather expected me to become a Naval Officer. Mum was open-minded about the whole thing and was more concerned about my happiness and achieving good 'O Level' results.

The time for the exams loomed ever nearer and I began to get a sense of urgency, I was not working hard enough at school and I certainly was not studying enough at home. I just couldn't motivate myself. I used to start studying with all good intentions but then my concentration seemed to wander on to other things. I knew I was not prepared! I felt bewildered and confused at my attitude, but also powerless to do anything about it.

Soon after taking my exams I left school knowing that I had not done particularly well, but remained optimistic that somehow the results would prove me wrong.

I was free at long last. I was free from books, lessons,

teachers and everything else. I was an adult, be it a very immature one, but an adult nevertheless!

During the last months at school I was doing a Saturday job at Jarrold's Department Store in Norwich. This enabled me to save some money towards a moped that I was planning to buy when I was 16. Saturday was now a day to look forward to, for one thing there was a female colleague at work who was rather a dish and also more often than not David and I would go clubbing. The night club we went to was called the Samson; we became regular clients and even found a source where we could purchase alcohol. So many a night after swigging back four or five barley wines (holding our nose while doing so) we entered the premises well inebriated!

The Samson was rather expensive, especially for drinks, so we used to buy one or two and make them last all night. Mostly we used to stand near the girl's toilets or on the stairways where we could make a right nuisance of ourselves with the opposite sex. The best time was during the Festive Season, because then we could grab girls as they walked past and try to kiss them. Even then sometimes all we would get was a mouthful of teeth if we forced them too much! These acts of boldness by me were still just a cover up because sometimes my bluff would be called and I would be left standing there unable to return conversation.

My self-confidence I thought, would grow with age, so at this stage although frustrated by it, it had not became a nagging problem. I had made up my mind on one thing though and that was the fact that I adored the opposite sex and thought about them all the while. All the time I spent at the Samson I only had one girl friend and that wasn't serious or even physical. I had the odd close encounter on the dance floor, but that was it.

My 16th birthday came and went and I bought my moped, it was a Honda Graduate of which I was extremely proud. David bought one as well, but his was second-hand and looked old compared to mine. We became friendly with another lad who had a brand new Honda 50, which looked and sounded like a small motorbike, his name was Derek.

It was not long before all three of us were going everywhere together on our machines and Derek became a friend and rival to me. Like me, he came from a broken home but his mother, a district nurse, had never remarried. She was a very emotional person and this unpredictability seemed at times to rub off on Derek. There were instances when he would treat me like a good mate and others, especially after spending time with David, when he would try to dominate me. I knew David was trying to create a confrontation between Derek and I so I made sure he damn sure he did not succeed, always giving back as good as I received. There was one night when we were all up at the Samson when Derek for no reason decided to kick me in the groin, this of course was very painful but I did not let it show and without hesitation retaliated with a kick of my own. This was a typical episode in my relationship with Derek, of course as usual I hated and feared confrontation with anyone but I would not give in and my strength of character saw me through as it had before and would again. There were good times with Derek and David, and being all adolescents we still got into trouble and had our fair share of laughs.

We had a period when we used to telephone people at random and pretend to be a DJ on radio and get the recipient to answer three questions with the promise of a prize if answered correctly. We had many variations on this theme and used to take great pleasure from practicing them.

Another time we noticed a young lad, who was under age, riding a moped around the village. I posed as a police sergeant from Wymondham on the phone to his father telling him it had come to our knowledge about his son and could he please proceed to the police station and explain why he was there. We later heard that his son had been charged with under age riding!

By now I was deeply engaged in my cycle speedway and it became my greatest interest. Come winter time, I felt a big hole in my life and could not wait for summer to come round again.

My exam results were disappointing but not unexpected; in fact, I only achieved one 'O Level' in mathematics and that I only just scrapped through. So there it was, my career was obvious I would join the Royal Navy as a rating not an officer. I did not see any reason to hang around, so I went to Norwich and enrolled at the Naval Careers Office.

During the weeks to follow, I took an entrants examination and had a medical test which I passed and then waited with more trepidation for my entry date. I had been told not to expect an early one. With this in mind I started a temporary full time job.

Mum and Tom had a friend who was manager of a wholesale food warehouse in Norwich, so they rang him and asked if there were any jobs going for me. Within a couple of weeks I had started in my new employment, Initially I worked in the office sorting out orders but soon progressed to become driver's mate which I quite enjoyed as I got to know the different delivery drivers and also to see different areas of East Anglia. During the winter, however, I was soon moved inside the warehouse where I made up orders for the different shops.

Working life was certainly different from school, and for the year I was working prior to entering the Navy I learnt many things. I learned the value of money, and about people and by the time I left I had aged more in that year than any other previous one.

NAVY DAYS

Soon after my 17th birthday I received my travel warrant. It had not really sunk in until it arrived, then I knew I was about to embark on the biggest adventure of my short life. The month was July and the year 1974, the big day was approaching fast, so I began to make preparations for leaving. One of the biggest wrenches was selling my cycle speedway bike. I had grown to love the sport and had even become quite good at it! During the last days I began to feel detached from reality and suddenly realised that the friends I had made over the last few years did not mean all that much to me. David and I had grown apart, and he was seeing a lot more of Derek than ever before. It made me aware that I was not leaving much behind.

Of course, my family was my main concern and especially Mum who I had never been apart from before. I had now learned that Tom had been moved again with his job, and he and Mum would be moving to Scotland. Sue would be staying in Norfolk - she had a boy friend and did not want to move, so she was to stay with friends in Wymondham, at least for a while. This was quite handy for her as she worked in a bank in the town. Dad was thrilled that I was joining the Royal Navy, but a little disappointed that it was not as an officer.

Along came the day of departure and the family were there to wave me off. I felt numb and seemed in a dream world as the train pulled out of the station. I was in half a mind to forget the idea and jump off the train as I felt the first pangs of homesickness engulf me.

I had a long journey ahead of me and assumed it would take most of the day. The West Country, where I was heading, meant I had to change in London which broke up the journey and also gave me an opportunity to meet Dad. We had lunch together and I listened to his enthusiastic conversation. Anyone would think it was him joining up, not me!

Nevertheless it was me and on leaving London the realisation of it all almost overwhelmed me. I was going to give it my best shot and not give in to these feelings of isolation.

On arrival at Plymouth, there was a reception committee where I and a few others were bundled into a lorry and driven to the ferry which would take us over the river to Torpoint. The clank of the chains was very distinctive and soon would become an all too familiar sound. From Torpoint the lorry travelled a further couple of miles until we pulled into an entrance and passed a sign saying HMS 'Raleigh'.

We were shown into a building, one of a row, where there were a few other lads waiting. It was very quiet, everyone seemed apprehensive which was very understandable - it was a large base and there were a lot of sailors everywhere.

Within an hour another lorry pulled up outside and out jumped 18 lads from Scotland, mainly Glasgow and what's more they all seemed to know each other. The silence was shattered; I had a terrible feeling that I had to spend the next six weeks with this rabble. I suddenly felt very homesick.

Things quietened down as a Chief Petty Officer made an entrance. He introduced himself and told us he would see us safely through the first week, after which, we would be moved across the base for basic training. He seemed a very nice man and told us that if anyone wished to leave they would be put on a train in the morning and nothing more would be said. The remainder would be required to sign a paper and commit themselves to the six weeks training. After supper we were all eager to pick the Chief's brains and find out all we could about the training. He really was a nice man and I thought that at least the first week would not be too bad. I went to bed that evening and was almost overcome by the feeling of loneliness and panic associated with homesickness.

I survived the night and woke up feeling a little better. One lad decided to go home and disappeared promptly leaving the rest of us to familiarise ourselves with each other and the surroundings.

After breakfast we were taken to the block opposite and asked to sign the paper after which we congregated back in our original building that we were now to call our mess. The Chief returned, but this time he carried a large stick which he promptly slammed down on the table and shouted for quiet. Everyone was stunned into silence, and I realised the honeymoon was over. We were now to address the Chief as Sir and in his presence to speak only when spoken to. Many other rules and conditions were laid down and the Chief told us, in no uncertain terms, about how we were expected to behave.

The first week at *Raleigh* was very busy and tiring - I was not used to getting up at 6.30am. We were taught how to look after our kit, the rudiments of marching, and the importance of cleanliness and hygiene, and most importantly the value of discipline.

By the end of the week everyone was shell-shocked, including myself, so much had been done and taught us, that we had not had any free time and certainly had not been allowed outside the base.

We were moved on, everyone was happy at the prospect. For one thing we were to be allowed leave and for another we no longer felt detached from the rest of humanity, we were now part of the base and able to mix with the other ratings.

Our new instructor was a Petty Officer but still commanded respect, at the same time he became our friend and adviser. Over the next 5 weeks we were taught to become proper sailors. The time passed too quickly and new friendships were made, most of the Scottish lads lost their initial prejudice and mellowed their aggressiveness becoming warmer and friendlier as each day passed. There were exceptions, including one who was an Englishman of around 28 years of age who sported a full beard and enjoyed nothing more than a good drinking session at the local pubs. Now this man, who was called John, had taken a dislike to me and consequently arriving back after a drinking session used to take great pleasure in tipping me out of bed. As I was in the top bunk this was no laughing matter. Night upon night I grew to expect this unpleasant occurrence and it was not long before it wore me down to such an extent that I could not take much more. Finally, I reached a point when I burst into tears and almost begged him to stop. My friends, realising my predicament, supported me and said enough was enough, where upon John got the message and ceased his nocturnal bullying.

During John's vindictive period, I never once thought about retaliating violently - he was so much bigger than I and so much older that it never crossed my mind. Subsequently, at a later date, after upsetting another person, John backed down at the threat of violence which made me think, in hindsight, what would have happened if I had retaliated.

The first 6 weeks were basic training and consisted of marching, swimming, safety and fire prevention as well as fire fighting expeditions and fitness building. All this culminated in tough scrutiny at the end to see who would progress onto phase two and seamanship training.

Night leave was now allowed, but only in uniform. So many of the lads, including myself, used to take nights out in either Torpoint or Plymouth when not on duty.

My love life still did not improve, not for the lack of trying though. My confidence with girls was still low and was becoming more and more troublesome to me, especially as some of the other lads boasted of their conquests which added to my frustration.

Drinking became my main pastime and I even accompanied John on occasions, most of the time we visited Torpoint and never ventured to Plymouth on the ferry.

Duties were many and varied and I enjoyed most of them, I gained a sense of importance especially doing night duty which often meant dressing up in full uniform and in the case of a ferry patrol wearing white belt and gaiters. Despite losing your right to leave whilst on duty, I used to take every task very seriously and I think this reflected the self-discipline I had gained from my military training. I grew to enjoy the discipline of *Raleigh* and wrongly expected everyone else to take it as seriously.

Nevertheless, comradeship blossomed and while you tended to go on night leave with the odd one or two mates you invariably ended up in a large group of fellow sailors. On one such occasion, a night out in Plymouth was arranged and a visit to the famous night club called

'Rooftops' was the destination. The venue was a well-known haunt for 'first-term' uniformed sailors, but it was also the scene of some fighting with the local yobbos.

The night I chose to go was a Friday and a group of us set off and had a couple of drinks in Torpoint before venturing across the ferry into Plymouth. Once there we visited another couple of bars before arriving at the disco around 10 o'clock. As soon as we entered the club I could detect an atmosphere of aggression. I felt uneasy all night and did not enjoy the occasion at all. However nothing happened inside, but as we left and congregated in the street there were local youths menacingly gathering in groups. Outside the club, the number of sailors was easily 2 to 1 against the locals and providing we stuck together there was safety in numbers. Unfortunately most of our brave servicemen decided to run for it, so I and those who were left had no choice but to do likewise.

After a couple of minutes it was like a battle scene, any sailor that was caught by the pursuing youths was set upon and quite brutally beaten. I came quite close to being attacked, but managed to evade capture by the skin of my teeth. After losing our pursuers, a couple of sailors and I went back through the gauntlet of youths to find our missing mates. The situation was still volatile and after a few more narrow escapes we came upon one victim who had been badly beaten and he needed help to walk. We helped him back to the ferry where there was comparative safety, and where the Naval Police were interviewing the shaken survivors of the night's escapades. It was not until everyone arrived back at base that the true circumstances of the evening were known.

Many sailors had to go to hospital with their injuries and many more needed some sort of treatment.

Looking back in retrospect I knew that if only the sailors had stuck together and had not run, then a lot of the injuries would not have happened.

Life went on and the 6 weeks initial training was over. Out of the 23 who started only 12 made it through to phase two and the seamanship training. I was one of the 12. The remnants of the original class were granted a week's leave to celebrate our passing phase one.

Mum and Tom now lived in Scotland, so I was issued with the appropriate travel warrant and donned my uniform and set off on a new adventure. Mum was very pleased to have her little boy back home and even Tom seemed pleased to see me. The week went very quickly, which was just as well because really there was nothing to do. I had no friends in Scotland and I felt like a fish out of water. One thing that was discussed was my future.

There was concern, especially expressed by Mum that I had no training in any trade and if I was to pursue seamanship training it was all well and good while I was in the Navy, but what if I left.

This question played on my mind most of the week and come the end of my leave - after much soul-searching - I decided that trade training would be a very useful thing to have. So I made up my mind to change branches to trainee electrician on my return to base.

As my train pulled out of Edinburgh station I gave Mum a final wave and I could see that she was in tears which nearly set me off as well! It had been very nice to see her again, and I realised that I would miss her very much!

Many things changed in phase two, out went most of the square bashing and incessant kit inspections, and in came tutoring on seamanship. I had put in my request to change to an electrician and was told that it would take some weeks; in the meantime I was to carry on as normal.

Also in phase two we did a lot more practical seamanship which involves learning to handle different types of boat, from lifeboats to sailing boats and even rowing boats. We had also been moved again, this time into a much more modern block which was much easier to keep clean and much warmer with up to date toilet facilities. Another major change was that we were allowed to wear civilian clothes when on leave from the base.

Everyone was now more relaxed and relationships which began in phase one became, if anything, much closer and permanent. I had become a well-liked and respected member of the class especially after entering the base's boxing competition and finishing runner-up in my weight division. Mainly because I had a bye through to the final.

I did not have any really close friends at this time, but did get on well with almost everybody and enjoyed some of the pranks the lads got up to. One that springs to mind is the time we carried a sleeping sailor outside, still tucked up in bed, and left him there all night.

After getting used to the new surroundings things settled down to as near normal as possible with a group of young sailors who lived together. A new pastime evolved in our living quarters which were strictly against the rules, namely taking part in séances. I dabbled in it a bit, but found it rather intense and frightening so I became a reluctant observer. One particular evening I was lying on my bunk reading, trying to ignore the proceedings, when the glass apparently spelt out my name unbeknown to me. Of course, when told about this

I freaked out and refused to join the circle but the glass became very persistent and after much persuasion I reluctantly joined the excited participants. Immediately I put my finger on the glass, the contact became less frantic and began to identify itself. It left me in no doubt that it was my Mum's brother who had died at the end of the last war. As the contact progressed it began to spell out a message but was interrupted by a cynic who decided enough was enough and started to disrupt matters by mocking and laughing at us. After that the contact became disturbed and seemed preoccupied with venting its anger on the cynic who, whenever close, immediately sent the glass haywire! Eventually the contact was lost. It was decided afterwards that no further experiments in the occult would take place. I was very relieved!

As I said things were more relaxed in phase two and the lads led an easy going life. It became more like a nine to five job and there were less duties to do, so more free time. My free time was spent in search of love; I was still looking for my first sexual encounter. My quest took me into Plymouth a lot more and I used to visit many pubs in the centre of town. Some of them had strippers and dancers which have always been a favourite. However, watching girls and chattering to them are completely different - one I found easy, the other hard. I was becoming more and more disillusioned and frustrated; it was as though the girls sensed this and shied away from me. My escape, once again, was drink and as the time progressed I spent more time drinking locally in Torpoint and decided that the right girl would come to me! Fate it was called, wasn't it?

Time was on my side I suppose although it passed quickly and it was not long until final exams and I was waiting to hear about my next posting.

One night whilst on duty around the canteen area I was wondering why the time was going so slowly when I noticed a sailor kicking a vending machine. I had met this particular lad before and as far as I was concerned he was a trouble-maker. So I approached him and told him to stop his violence towards the machine or I would report him. Without warning he tried to throw a punch at me, however, because of his reputation I was half expecting it. After a few seconds of scuffling I managed to overpower him and told him that I would definitely report him to the Duty Petty Officer, and then released him. He ran off and I was left trying to compose myself and stop shaking before going to see my superior officer. On arrival at the office, I was summoned in and told that my behaviour had been completely out of order and I was lucky not to go on report. It was obvious that my assailant had beaten me to it and had told a pack of lies. I tried to tell my side of the story, but the Duty Petty Officer would not listen and made me apologise for my actions. I could not believe what was happening, but decided to let the matter rest.

Apart from that one incident my remaining time at *Raleigh* passed quietly and it was then final examinations and Passing Out. Passing Out is what all servicemen do when they finish their training. It involves dressing in your best uniform and doing a march past a high ranking officer on the parade ground. Some sailors also receive awards and I would have received one for achieving 100% in my seamanship exams, but I was changing to a trade so that honour went to John who also obtained full marks.

Drafting followed immediately and most of my classmates were being sent to Portsmouth to learn about

Sonar, Radar or Gunnery while I received my posting to HMS 'Collingwood' which was at Fareham in Hampshire. I was to learn about Electronics!

Farewells were said and Good Luck to All as we made our ways to our next destination. I felt a certain sadness leaving Torpoint and Cornwall - it is a lovely area with beautiful scenery - but, as I had already learned life must go on, and so ended another period in my life.

HMS 'Collingwood' was the largest shore base in the country and, as I walked through the main gate, it certainly looked huge. The parade ground was twice the size of the one at *Raleigh* and the buildings surrounding it seemed never ending. I was directed to the new entry block and found it already inhabited by most of my new classmates. There was not such a Scottish presence in this new bunch although they all seemed to know each other, which was understandable as they had done their basic training together. I later found out, that they had only been in for six weeks against my fifteen, so were not yet allowed to wear civilian clothes on leave, whereas I was, this created a certain amount of envy.

Comradeship, as I had found at *Raleigh*, was evident at *Collingwood* and it did not take long to get familiarised with the lads and I settled down quickly. One thing I noticed from the start though was the big reduction in discipline, the base was much easier going than *Raleigh* and I found it hard to adjust. There was a certain amount of security before, but now everything seemed so lax. We did not even have a class instructor and had to rely on ourselves to get to lessons on time. After a week we were moved into another modern block. This was to be our permanent home for the duration. Although there were four to a room it was not completely sectioned off as there was an open corridor running along the side, so there were lots of comings and goings throughout the day and night. Although we were separated only by walls some people thought it was closed off enough not to be heard. They made a racket at night, so it was not long before I laid down the law about the noise and thus started to get another reputation. No one ever called my bluff - it was just as well because I do not know to this day whether I would have backed up my words.

Simon was a lad who had followed from *Raleigh.* I had known him before but not all that well, now at *Collingwood* we became good friends and spent a lot of time together. We used to go to Southampton at least once a week to the ice-rink. It was a good place to meet girls, and sailors used to frequent it regularly. The added attraction to me was that it had a bar which overlooked the rink, so you could eye the talent whilst having a drink. There was also a Disco most nights which created a good atmosphere and even now when I hear 'Come up and see me, make me smile' by Steve Harley and Cockney Rebel it takes me back to some very good nights at the Southampton ice-rink.

I did pull a couple of girls at this time but took it too seriously and paid the price, so my virginity stayed intact for a while longer! However, these few weeks were good times on which I look back with affection.

Back at base, I was getting more and more disillusioned. I found the work hard to get to grips with, and the lack of discipline amongst my classmates was winding me up. I became unhappy and frustrated.

To help cheer myself up I bought a motorbike, a brand new Honda CB200 and often took myself off on expeditions around the Hampshire countryside. This worked for a time, but soon I slipped back into unhappiness which I decided was due to my lack of a relationship. Whatever I thought the reason, I could not seem to shake it off and turned more and more to drinking as a means of escape. I remember after one particular session walking back to the dormitory. I crossed the huge parade ground, with the wind blowing a gale, thinking how lonely and isolated I felt. Yet I felt exhilarated by the experience and felt I was not alone and that something or somebody was with me to help face a battle that was yet to come. A battle that I could not even begin to know the intensity of.

I started to attend the church every Sunday thinking maybe I could find some answers there, but my restlessness continued. I failed to gain any answers except that I believed in God, but I had my own way of recognising this and going to church was not it.

Whatever was causing the problem my work was beginning to suffer? I found it hard to concentrate and increasingly my thoughts would wander off and I slipped into my own little world. I had lost interest in my career! This, of course, became another worry for me.

Inevitably things came to a head. It was a March afternoon and as usual the class lined up in rank and file after lessons waiting for the class leader to be appointed to march us back to our accommodation block. Class leaders at *Collingwood* were a fiasco, a different one elected everyday, while at *Raleigh* one was appointed permanently so within a short time he gained respect, if he was worth his salt.

Meanwhile, this particular afternoon the biggest waster in the whole class was elected, so before even setting off I knew the march would be a shambles and if seen by a superior officer would result in trouble. Sure enough, it was as I predicted and everyone was marching

- if you could call it marching - at almost running speed, all except my file which was at the proper pace. The appointed class leader told us to close up but I ignored him, so therefore my file stayed with me. With that the class leader said he would report me if I did not obey his commands. That was the last straw for me, so I just told him to shove it and walked off and made my own way back.

The following day I learned that I had been put on Commander's report, which meant that I would have to appear in front of the Commander in a few days. Ironically the same day I was appointed class leader and had a dreadful time controlling the men while marching back from class. They obviously now had it in for me and did their utmost to misbehave which was noticed by a Petty Officer, who immediately held me responsible and told me to report to the main gate that evening. Still not believing what was happening, I arrived at the main gate at the designated time expecting another report. After a long conversation with the Petty Officer concerned he decided to let me off with a warning as he had heard that I was already in trouble. My relationship with my classmates deteriorated further and this time I was just glad that my room mates gave me their support and, along with help from Simon, made life tolerable.

The day of the Commander's Table arrived and I was appointed a Lieutenant to defend me. After reading up on my case he advised me that the only way to proceed was to plead guilty to the charge. This was against everything I had planned, and I had prepared myself for a long drawn out defence. I was innocent and did not want to give in to the bastards who had put me there in the first place.

The Lieutenant was very persistent, and

persuasive and began to wear me down, he even suggested that my 'pig headedness' would get me into even more trouble. Against my better judgement I relented and pleaded guilty and received 10 days all leave stopped and 10 days working in the kitchens. To this day I regret pleading guilty and know that apart from making more enemies I would have won my case and escaped the unjust punishment meted out to me.

The animosity between a certain classmate and I remained and we nearly came to blows once or twice, this only went towards intensifying my growing disillusionment with my life in the Navy. I could not help but think that I should have remained a seaman and pursued a career without a trade, because the way my class work was progressing it would be an uphill struggle to become qualified anyway.

I began to think more and more about leaving. I was not yet 18 so had not officially signed a contract and if I did not try now it would soon be too late.

While considering my options we were sent to sea for a couple of days. This experience made up my mind for me. I was very adverse to the sleeping conditions on board ship. They were very cramped and I suffered from claustrophobia, which I reported to my Commanding Officer.

On returning to *Collingwood* I put in my request for a discharge and while waiting for news pondered on my decision and future.

I had no idea what I was going to do in Civvy Street, but hoped at least that I would feel happier about myself. Once again I appeared at the Commander's Table but was immediately passed on to the Captain, as it was a very important, decision.

The Captain's Table was just as formal as the

Commander's and after hearing the reasons for my request he surprisingly gave a response straight away. Discharged, unsuitable for further training! I was stunned - it had all been so easy and quick, and final. I could not reverse it now even if I had wanted to, and the word unsuitable stuck in my mind. Had my service record been that bad?

Nevertheless, I was out and within a week of the decision, after a few goodbyes, I rode through the main gate for the last time and without looking back accelerated away.

It was April 1975; I had been in the Royal Navy almost, 10 months. It had been a career that started so promisingly at *Raleigh* and slowly deteriorated after my arrival at *Collingwood.* I hoped and prayed that I had made the right decision, and looked to my future with apprehension!

THE SEARCH FOR A CAREER

My first destination was Witham. I had arranged to stay with my Granny and Granddad for a few days and this enabled me to see Dad at the same time. As I rolled up on my motorbike it looked as if nothing had changed, the quiet little close where they lived still had the familiar feeling and my Grandparents greeted me in their unique, warm and friendly way.

I settled in quickly and soon relaxed into the routine of life. I was soon pottering about the garden with Granddad and running errands for Granny. I knew though that boredom would set in once the novelty had worn off. With this in mind I rode round to Dad's when I could. It was good to see him again although I could tell that he was upset about me leaving the Navy. Hazel was her same moody self, so I did my best to keep out of her way! Dad tried to persuade me to come and stay with them for a while but I would have none of it. I was not going to risk being with Hazel at this time.

The big talk in the family at this time was the impending marriage of my sister, Sue, to her boy friend Mark. The happy day was to be in June, so there was not much point in me going to Scotland before the big day as the ceremony was to be in Norfolk.

I survived a couple of weeks in Witham, and then decided to go up to Norfolk as I had an invitation from Mum's friend to stay for a short while. I said my goodbyes to Granny and Granddad, and Dad and remarked that I would see them all again at the wedding. With that I rode off into the sunset.

As it happened it was not the end of the day, it was a bright, sunny May morning and I was in no real hurry.

It takes about 2 hours to reach Wymondham from Witham normally, but on this particular day it took a great deal longer. I suppose I was about half way and I was riding through a small village doing around thirty miles an hour. When, without warning, a car pulled out of a garage straight into my path. It all happened so quickly that I did not have time to take evasive action and barely had time to brake, so I ploughed into the side of the car. Releasing my grip on the handlebars I cart wheeled clean over the car and landed in a heap on the other side. Initially I was a bit stunned so I gingerly got to my feet and realised that I was not hurt, in fact all I had was a graze on my leg.

Relieved at the outcome I went over to inspect my machine. This, as I was afraid, was a different story. It looked a mess, the front forks were very twisted and there were a lot of scratches and dents on the front end, it was clearly unridable.

The driver of the car was a young lady who was very shocked and apologetic. So I decided that there would be nothing to gain by being angry with her, although I was not feeling exactly happy about the situation. We exchanged insurance details and other necessities and discussed the facts about the accident, with which I was quite happy. A couple of witnesses at the garage agreed with us, so all I had to do was to get to Wymondham.

After a few calls, a motorcycle dealer from Norwich agreed to come and pick up my bike and to do the repairs. It was 2 hours before he arrived and by that time I was well and truly fed up!

I eventually arrived at my destination at teatime and it soon started to dawn on me that for the next few days I was trapped where I was and even if I wanted to leave, I couldn't. So I hoped my stay would be a happy one, for my feelings of discontentment were returning and I only hoped that I could prevent myself getting depressed again.

There is not much to tell about my life in the time prior to the wedding. The friends I stayed with were also giving a temporary home to Sue. She worked in the local bank so was out most of the day, whereas up until I had my motorbike back I was more or less restricted to the house. Things were made much easier once I had my transport back and I took full advantage of my newly regained freedom. The days passed and the wedding loomed. Sue started to get cold feet which I thought was only natural, and by the time the big day arrived she needed a lot of reassurance that she was doing the right thing.

The day itself went smoothly, first the wedding and then the reception. The wedding was held at Wymondham Abbey, just outside Norwich, while the reception was at Hethersett. All our family were there and this included Dad and Hazel who had behaved herself remarkably well. A good time was had by all with plenty to eat and drink, the later being tested to the limit by Hazel!

Mum and Tom stayed in Norfolk for a week before returning to Scotland once the celebrations were over. I came to the decision that I would join them and look for work from that base. I had had enough of living out of a suitcase. At this time in my life I still regarded home as living with Mum, and most of my possessions were with her. It would give me time to sort myself out, I hoped!

Once again, I set off on my travels, I had never been such a distance on my bike before and did not realise how much of an endurance test it would be, but I made it and was glad to be home.

Mum was pretty good; she did not nag me too much about getting a job, certainly initially. As the days passed I started to buy trade newspapers and magazines looking for ideas. I still did not know what I wanted to do for a career. Even at the tender age of 18 my main objective was to get into a relationship, not just physical but much deeper than that. It was becoming an obsession and it made me miserable. Nevertheless, my priority was a job and I had to knuckle down and get one.

One day I was looking through the different advertisements in my growing pile of literature when I noticed one offering work in the licensed trade in London. Accommodation was provided and no fee required as the commission would be paid by the employer. It was an agency, and I immediately telephoned them for further information. Satisfied with what I heard I told them I would be down there the following week, so that was that!

The journey down south was just as hard and laborious as the one up. I had arranged to stay with Dad for one night to provide a base for me close to London. I was sure I could put up with Hazel for a single night, and besides I did not have much choice! The night passed without too much incident and I even enjoyed the different company for a change. Dad, as usual, gave me some advice on the licensed trade - he had had a lot of experience in that line with Hazel - and he liked a tipple himself.

I arrived at the agency at around midday the following morning and was surprised to see how many clients they had already waiting, including some very tasty young ladies. By the afternoon some of us were sent to work at a restaurant as trainee waiters, but I am afraid that it did not last long for me. I was like a fish out of water and the boss soon became fed up and early the next day I was unceremoniously sacked. So I landed back at the agency for another post, preferably not in a restaurant. I was offered a position as full-time barman at a pub, which seemed a bit more to my liking. So I said I would take it and arrived there ready to start the evening session.

The pub was called The Crown and Anchor and was situated near Euston Station. The landlord or should I say manager was a friendly guy called Bobby Cox, who I later found out was an alcoholic. His wife, Dawn, was much more moody and had a nasty temper if crossed. She had an attractive face, but her figure was not much to write home about possibly because of giving birth to two children. She had a lover, a rather nasty piece of work, who stayed in the background and never entered the premises, well almost never! Bobby, of course, knew about the man and did not seem to mind, except that he was shit scared of him but so were a lot of people. There was also a barmaid, an Irish lass Eileen, who was a pleasant enough person, but again she had an unpleasant side when upset. Eileen and I became friends as the time went by, maybe because I showed her some respect and did not upset her. Also because I never said anything about her and her boy friend's noisy lovemaking that kept me awake some nights.

My bedroom was next to Eileen's and had a door straight into hers just like some hotels. It was just as well that I did not really fancy her because her boy friend once told us that he had strung a piece of cotton across the doorway! He, like a lot of other customers in the pub, demanded respect. It was in a rough area and most of them were in a different league to me, and that's how I kept it. I was not and never would be a violent person. The Crown and Anchor was a pub with two sides: lunchtimes it was very much used by office workers; while in the evenings the locals considered it their pub and used to congregate up one particular end and keep an eye on whoever came through the door.

It took a while for me to be accepted, so in the evenings when around the locals I did my best to keep them happy without being too submissive, while keeping Bobby happy by being efficient at my other tasks. I soon found out that there was a lot more to being a barman than meets the eye, especially amongst such a volatile clientele as we had. You had to learn when a conversation was for your ears, and when it was not, behave accordingly. After a while I got to know other locals and spent a lot of my time chatting with them. I think the others accepted me, realised I was not a danger and let me get on with it.

Lunchtimes were more relaxed affairs and I soon started to strike up acquaintances with various people. I remember one particular man who often used to buy me drinks and chat while I was working. He seemed very ordinary at the time, so ordinary in fact that when he asked me to come for drink one night I thought why not he might introduce me to a few females.

So, there it was, one evening I met up with him and went to the Earls Court area to a few pubs. Little did I know initially that they were gay pubs and that my so called friend was also gay and fancied me! Of course, when it dawned on me what was happening, I told him that I was not interested in him and liked girls. This he seemed to accept and conceded defeat without turning nasty. Nevertheless the memory of that night stays with me to this day, some of the places he took me to were very intimidating to a naive 18-year-old and they contained many varieties of people from all walks of life. If anything good came of it, it was the fact that it served to strengthen my own sexuality and made me realise I should never be so quick to judge people again.

Apart from that incident I barely ventured out from the pub, mainly because I could not afford it and also did not have a mate to go out with. My main pastime was still drinking and often finished bar sessions, especially in the evenings, three sheets to the wind!

Bobby used to run up big bar bills and sort them out before the next stocktaking. There were various ways he used to settle them, but mainly he would to go up the cash and carry and buy bottles of spirits and pour them into the optics in the pub, until he guessed he had covered his bill. This was sometimes as high as £300. This, like many other things, I used to turn a blind eye to.

As I became more experienced, more and more of the workload rested on my shoulders. I used to do all the bottling up and the cellar work as well. I did not mind very much as it kept me on the right side of Bobby. One thing he let me do which he was not too keen on, was allowing me to wheel my motorbike inside the pub every night to stop it getting vandalised. I also had the odd bottle of lager off the shelf.

The time went quickly, and I found I was fairly contented. The only thing that got me down was the now usual lack of female company. There was one part-time barmaid who I quite fancied but she had a boy friend, so did not pursue it apart from making my feelings known. I later found out that if I had pursued the issue I may have had a result. Another one that got away!

Christmas was looming and I started to get restless. I thought about my loneliness and felt sorry for myself. I could not go home for Christmas, which was just as well because Mum and Tom were to come down to Norfolk and we were all to spend it at Sue's house.

Christmas Eve at the pub was hectic and for once there was a mixture of office workers and locals. A recipe for disaster was in the air and I could see it was only a matter of time before tempers erupted, and I feared for the safety of some of the innocents. It all started well with people in festive spirit, but as the day wore on and more and more locals came in the atmosphere changed.

It was late afternoon when the trouble started. One of the locals had taken a dislike to a stranger and decided to smash a glass in his face. I never actually saw the incident but there was plenty of blood around, and women screaming and yelling. Bobby, although worse for drink as usual, took charge of the situation and decided to shut the pub. So everyone, including the locals were persuaded to leave. That was my first taste of what real violence was like and it sickened me and as far as I could see it was all caused by people having too much to drink and thinking they are something they are not. I knew from then on my days at the Crown and Anchor were numbered.

I bottled up before I left for Norfolk because I knew it would not have been done otherwise. The journey was a good one and only took me two and a half hours, so I arrived with enough time to celebrate down at the local pub.

Everybody seemed in a festive mood. All except for my sister's husband which put a damper on things.

Mum and Tom were not pleased with his attitude and threatened to return home if things did not improve. They did slightly, but come Christmas Day we spent it hardly having a single drink. The host's attitude left a lot to be desired, so once again we congregated at the local pub.

Boxing Day was not much different apart from the food, Sue did us proud! Everybody was pleased that this particular festive season was behind them. After saying my farewells I rode off back to London feeling strangely sad. I had felt that way a few times by then. I could not understand why, but wondered whether it was to do with the strange loneliness I felt.

Things were the same back at the pub except for the fact that I found it harder to relax and be at ease with the people around me. As New Year came and went I began to notice the tensions a lot more than before and felt ill at ease with anyone who was the least bit aggressive. This was quite a number considering the clientele we entertained.

One evening, while Bobby was out and the bar was quiet, one of the locals walked in. This man had a reputation for violence and had been known to possess a gun, so I was very aware of the potential for trouble. It was not long before I established he had been rowing with his wife, whom he adored, so he was on a very short fuse and was in the mood for drinking. He stayed about an hour then decided to visit another watering hole, so I breathed a sigh of relief when he left. The rest of the evening was quiet enough so I closed the bar promptly and started clearing up.

As the last customer left and I was washing the remaining glasses, the man in question returned and was obviously blind drunk. He started to repeatedly push the door open, but did not venture in. So I left him to get on with it while I finished up. Unfortunately the pet Alsatian started barking at him, so without thinking I shouted at the excited animal to stop. Without hesitation the door was kicked open and the bar flap, which was covered in glasses, was thrust aside and I was slammed by my neck across the counter. By the look in his eyes he wanted to kill someone and I was petrified. So I just froze and explained that I was shouting at the dog and not at him.

After a couple of minutes he relaxed his hold on me and disappeared out the door. I do not think I have ever been so frightened in my life, and even after he apologised the next day my love for the pub trade was severely damaged, particularly that pub.

All through the six months that I was working at the Crown and Anchor I took pity on the Alsatian, most of its days were spent down in the cellar and it was lucky to be taken out just once a day. I took it out when I could and gave it my affection. It was so docile and it saddened me the way it was treated by its owners. By the time the day came to leave I had become very attached to him and he was the one regret I left behind.

It was a messy way to leave, but nevertheless the timing was right. In the final weeks I had, as I have already mentioned become more and more unhappy and a lot of things were coming to a head. My last evening happened to be my evening off and I decided to have a drink in the bar. There was one of the young local lads sitting there when I arrived. He was about my age and had been goading me for a long time about how tough he was and was for ever asking me outside for a fight. I had always declined the invitation, but this particular night he kept on and on and was slowly winding me up. In the end I became so agitated I thought it best to go upstairs and leave him to it.

Unfortunately Dawn was at home and she started pulling me up on a few things that she did not like about me. So in return, being still in a bad mood, I returned the compliment and had a go at her! I think the part when I called her a cow was probably the last straw, so with that she told me I was sacked and to get my things and leave immediately. I did what she said as I had had enough, although I became upset because of all the things I had done for them, especially for Bobby who was not there at the time. I managed to find a bed for the night at a friendly customer's place, to whom I was extremely grateful.

In the morning I rang Mum and told her I would be coming home, so leaving my thanks I got on my bike and set off for Scotland once more.

The journey home was again very long and arduous; it was a February day and very cold. By the time I arrived I was frozen stiff and had to be helped off my bike. It was evening and dark, and I had spent a lot of the journey thinking about my future but once I was warm again fatigue swept over me so all I wanted to do was sleep.

I woke up the next morning determined not to be a burden to my Mum and Tom and to look for a job straight away. I was lucky, within a few days I managed to find work in a brick factory which was situated in a small village called Whitecross. This was only 3 miles from home, home being as I have not mentioned it before, Linlithgow.

The job entailed shift work, a week of early shifts, seven in the morning until three in the afternoon alternating with a week of late shifts, three in the afternoon to eleven at night. The work was nearly always physically easy and not the least bit taxing on the mind, but at the same time not boring.

The first thing I noticed was the number of women workers in the factory and the type of language they used. They were worse than any of the men and it certainly opened my eyes. I had never experienced anything like it before and never heard the like again! Apart from the 'effing and blinding', when you got to know them they were quite nice people. If you had the opportunity to meet them in their homes, you found that they never uttered one swear word and their homes were immaculate.

As I settled into my job, I got to know many people and was interested to learn that most of the workers were related to one another, and what's more the majority lived in Whitecross. I began to assume that as it was such a tight knit community I would have trouble making friends, but this was not so. As I look back I can safely say that I have never had, before or since, so many friends as I had during my time in Scotland.

Most of my mates used to use a pub, about half way between home and work, called The Bridge Inn. It was a lively place and used to have live music at weekends, so I spent quite a few evenings drinking there. When I first went to The Bridge or any other pub for that matter, I kept a low profile to start off with because I was well aware that I was the only Englishman amongst so many Scots. I need not have worried; I never met any prejudice and was largely accepted.

It was up at The Bridge that I met Karen. She was very attractive and I was more or less hooked from day one. She lived in Whitecross with her parents, so was only a 10 minute ride away. Our romance lasted two weeks before she started to avoid me. There seemed to be no real reason why she did this except that she was married to someone else within three months.

Nevertheless, I had fallen in love and was left hurt and frustrated by it, and what's more my virginity stayed intact!

The frustration seemed to stay with me long after time had cured the hurt, but I did my best to suppress it. Unfortunately, it came out one night and nearly got me in deep trouble. I was in The Bridge one Friday with a couple of mates when we got talking to a couple of girls. They were friendly enough, and at the end of the evening they allowed us to walk them home. On the way I decided to put my arm round one of them, but she shook it off, which annoyed me so I put it back and pulled her towards me. She then became very aggressive and told me to leave her alone. Very annoyed at her behaviour I said that she was an ugly old cow and I would not touch her with a barge pole and walked off.

By the next day the affair was all over the village, followed by a rumour that the girl's father was looking for me. I was still annoyed by the girl's attitude and believed I was justified in doing what I did. But after seeing my mates again and getting their opinion I began to realise that I had gone too far and maybe an apology was in order. I did apologise to the girl, who reluctantly accepted it, but I still felt hard done by and still thought that her attitude left a lot to be desired. Not many days after the incident my motorbike was vandalised outside The Bridge, whether the two incidents were connected or not I shall never know.

Soon things started to settle down again and work carried on as normal. I started to notice a lady at work. She was a good 10 years older than me and not exactly an oil painting, but there was something about her that attracted me. To this day I do not know what, because normally I am very fussy. Nevertheless, I pursued her and eventually asked her out and to my amazement she said, 'yes'! I took her out for a drink once, and then told her that I would take her out on my motorbike the next time we met. It was a warm early summer's evening and I took her into the countryside which she seemed to enjoy. We came to a meadow with a surrounding wall and gate which I promptly rode through and turned off the engine.

My first time was not exactly passionate, but my partner was very experienced and seemed to want to get it over with as quickly as possible. I was in a daze as I rode home and felt exhilarated. I had sampled the physical side of love and was hooked on it and would certainly try it again! I was 19 years of age and had lost my virginity at long last!

She did not want to know me after that despite all my efforts, so I put it down to experience. When I got over her I realised what she had done for me and felt a sense of gratitude and warmth to her.

My time in Scotland was to be cut short. Tom had another transfer, this time to London, and it was only a matter of weeks before he started. Mum asked me what I would do, stay in Scotland or would I move down to London? It was not a hard decision, I knew that my destiny was not in Scotland and I would never find true happiness there!

Recently I had started to think about fate and destiny and realised that something special was waiting for me somewhere, whether it be fame or fortune or just simple happiness. I became more and more pre-occupied with these thoughts and would dream that one day I would be happy and my feelings of sadness would be gone for ever.

Mum and Tom moved down to London early to look for a house and generally organise things. They already had a buyer for the property in Linlithgow, so the furniture was put in storage and I went to stay with friends of the family. The idea being that I would pack up shop when everything was finalised.

I continued to work but soon found the so-called friends of the family became very unfriendly and began to find fault with everything I did or did not do. After a couple of weeks I was made to feel distinctly unwelcome and decided to look for digs. The day I left they could not get rid of me quick enough and I'll always remember her using the Hoover and banging it against my bedroom door early that morning. They probably disinfected my room once I was gone! But gone I was, and I spent the rest of my time in Scotland in digs living with an old lady near Whitecross, which being close to my workplace was ideal!

During this time I kept in constant touch with Mum via the telephone and eventually at the end of August, having missed the hot summer of 1976 (the weather in Scotland was not that good) Mum told me that they were moving into a house in Bisley, near Woking in Surrey, and that I could join them at anytime. With this news I handed in my notice at work and at my digs and made my preparations for my departure. I went for a farewell drink with my mates and promised to keep in touch, as you do, and had my motorbike serviced for the long journey south. Early one Saturday morning I slipped away and left behind another life!

The house was newly built and was detached, with four

bedrooms. Being situated on an unfinished building site there was a lot of activity and even the road was unsurfaced. The first thing I did when I arrived was to sell my motorbike; having passed my driving test in Scotland I now wanted a car. Scanning the ads in the local newspaper I became interested in a Cortina, so wasting no time I persuaded Mum and Tom to take me to see it. We went and it was a good clean, white car with a pale green stripe down each side. I liked it and bought it, so I had wheels and now all I needed was a job!

It was not easy, good jobs were not easy to find, unemployment was high and I still had no idea of what career I wanted to pursue. The general feeling of unhappiness still haunted me, but I put that down to two things. Firstly my lack of a career and secondly the lack of a girl friend. My priority was a job and so I became less choosey and looked for anything, within reason. I finally found work more or less on my doorstep. One day, about three weeks after moving in, Mum suggested I see the foreman on the site where I lived. So I trudged over and learned that they wanted a ground worker and I could start almost immediately. I accepted the job and was told that the duties would involve digging, concreting, drain laying and general fetching and carrying for the tradesmen on the site.

As the starting day came around little did I realise that I was about to start a career that would span more than 10 years and give me duties that I could only imagine at that time. A career that would take me from the very bottom, nearly to the top - and also a career that I would grow to hate.

THE STORM CLOUDS GATHER

It was a dirty job and physically demanding, most of my workmates were Irish which I later found was quite common in that type of work. But they were a good bunch and all had a good sense of humour, which certainly made a difference in that working environment. One thing I noticed was my lack of stamina when it came to the demanding jobs like concreting. I first wondered if smoking was the reason, but then realised that a lot of the others smoked and were not affected. Perhaps it was down to all the heartburn I had been experiencing at that time. Whatever it was, if it became worse, I would have to go to the doctors.

The best part of the day was breakfast time when the mess man would prepare different meals for the lads. A few would have a cooked breakfast and one particular worker was partial to steak. He was the drain man and spent most of his time down manholes, but always seemed reluctant about washing his hands. When asked about this, he said it added to the flavour of the food! I always enjoyed a couple of boiled eggs with freshly baked bread and butter.

There were a lot of tradesmen on the site including, of course, bricklayers. The leader of the gang was nicknamed 'Mad Mitch', who when upset used to foam at the mouth and generally throw his weight around. It was our job to keep the tradesmen happy, but it was very difficult to keep 'Mad Mitch' content and there were many times when he had a saliva problem! One other tradesman who was prominent on the site was the roofer, his name was Keith, and he used to keep the men happy by showing them pornographic movies. So many nights I was late home because of Keith's entertainment; it used to be a very popular part of the day. On no account did I let on to Mum why I was sometimes late in the evenings. I always said I was doing overtime! Apart from the film shows, Keith and I soon became friends and he being only a couple of years older seemed to have a lot in common with me, however I lost temporary touch with him when he moved to a different site.

I was given a sort of promotion after a few weeks. I became the Dumper Driver, which was a very responsible position! The machine was a four wheel drive which had a huge bucket on the front and could go virtually anywhere. I used to enjoy riding about all day and felt a sense of importance driving such a big machine, and I parked it outside our home when I went home for lunch.

The work on my home site lasted only three months. After that the gang moved to another site. I was asked whether I wanted to go with them, but I decided to look for something more local. There were plenty of building jobs advertised, so I was very optimistic of finding work.

My social life at this time used to entail using the local pub, which was called the Hen and Chickens. Unfortunately there were few females that used it, so my love life was back to normal, namely non-existent! I used to go out most evenings for a couple of hours. One reason being that Tom was so stroppy most of the time, and had a habit of treating me like a four-year-old, which was a shame because he could be one of the nicest people around when in a good mood. Mum was aware of his moods but used to stick up for him the best she could, although she sympathised with me and suggested

I get an evening bar job, which I did!

Being experienced in bar work I soon settled in. The pub in question, called The Nags Head, was only a couple of miles away so it only took five minutes by car. The landlord was an ex-policeman and at first seemed to be a nice person, but as time wore on he showed his true colours! It was not a particularly busy pub so became boring on the couple of evenings I worked and as for women, forget it! However, initially it was a good little job and I decided to stay, and stay I did!

Little did I know that my social life was to be changed by my next job. I found it in the local paper; it caught my eye because it was local work within the building trade. It was also normal working hours which would mean that I could keep my evening bar job. Again it was a labouring job, but this time for a small local building firm which had just started a two-year contract at the nearby Mental Hospital called Brookwood. Brookwood Hospital was a big place, situated in Knaphill, about a mile from my home. The part I worked in was the boiler room which was being renovated, so there were welders and fitters on the site as well. My foreman, who was called Bill, was a big guy of about fifty who was a very skilled man. All the time I was there he demonstrated all aspects of the building trade from brick laying and plastering to drain laying and steel fixing (laying out steel reinforcing for concrete). Everything he did, he did well and took great pride in his work. He also believed in giving value for money so there was not much time for messing about, he kept everybody on their toes!

The work was hard and physical like my previous experience in the building trade and I did not particularly enjoy it, but it kept me reasonably fit and paid for my car and keep with a little bit over for beer. The thing that made it harder was the incessant heartburn I kept suffering mostly after lunch. As time went by it became worse and I knew it was nearly time to see a doctor, but at that time I was making do with indigestion tablets.

At this time, shortly after celebrating my 20th birthday in 1977, I was saddened to hear the news of the death of my Grandma in Essex. Apparently she died in her sleep, but looking back she was in her eighties so had quite a good, long life. Nevertheless, it upset me because she was good to me and I will always look back on her with affection.

Dad was philosophical about his mother's death and did not seem to be too affected by it, but he was never one to show his feelings. We all met up at the funeral and it was good to see all the family together again. Since moving to Surrey I had not seen Dad for some time and was interested to see if Hazel had mellowed towards me. She appeared just the same, except that she was drinking more than ever and still apparently had mood swings. She still did nothing to endear herself to me. Dad was forever trying to build bridges between myself and Hazel without much success. I could not help remembering how she treated me as a child.

Granddad being younger than Grandma was not suited to a life as a widower and was clearly affected by it, but within two years he had another companion and carried on living a contented life.

As I mentioned earlier my social life was in for a change with my job at Brookwood Hospital. Up until then I had been content to use The Hen and Chickens as my main watering hole, but within a few weeks of working there it was suggested that I use the Hospital Social Club. I was persuaded by one of the fitters on site about the advantages and arranged to meet him up there one evening. From then on I attended the club regularly and it became my main social haunt.

The attraction of the club was obvious compared to the pub. Firstly a lot of nurses used it, secondly the beer was cheaper and thirdly there was usually entertainment at weekends. My face soon became well known up there and I soon had regular drinking partners, mostly men a lot older than myself. It was at this time when, without realising it, I was tending to shy away from people my own age, feeling more comfortable with my elders and lacking the personality to mix with my peers (people my own age wanted more laughs).

One evening I was introduced to a nurse about my age and bought her a couple of drinks and actually relaxed for a change, finding I was getting on well with her. As the night wore on I developed the impression that she was only out for a good time, which was a shame because I liked her.

At the end of the evening, receiving an invitation to her room (most of the nurses lived in the hospital grounds), I thought I was in for a good evening. However, after a bit of a kiss and cuddle I tried my luck only to be rebuked. So, feeling frustrated again, I decided to get up and leave. So, with my tail between my legs, I left abruptly!

The following evening, I was sitting chatting in my normal place (near the bar), when who should walk in but my old mate Keith the roofer. He joined my company, and in answer to my question, told me that he used the social club because he was married to one of the nurses. After a while the nurse from the previous

evening walked in with a friend. I immediately told Keith about her and he replied that she was his wife, but told me not to worry because they were separated.
He then went into detail about why they were estranged and said that she had caught him in bed with another woman, and would not forgive him. He also said that she no longer trusted men and certainly would on no account have a one night stand! I was gutted at this revelation and realise that I had blown my first chance of a real relationship. I consequently tried to apologise for my previous behaviour but the damage could not be repaired, and I was left kicking myself for quite a while.

Most of my time was spent at the hospital now, in one capacity or another and I got to know many of the characters there. There was one old boy who I sometimes drank with called Charlie. He was a right character, as far as I could make out he had seen and done everything and always had a story to tell, whether it was the same one or a different one. There were also two German blokes who had apparently served in the war. They both seemed the right age and one was even rumoured to be an ex-SS soldier. The people I got to know were many and varied and most of them were nice people, although there were the odd few that I did not much care for.

My face became well known around the place and this also made work a bit more enjoyable. My duties, as I have indicated, were different from day to day. Most of the early work was situated in or around the boiler house itself.

One day I was inside removing old putty from the large and numerous windows, when something extraordinary happened. I was working up a ladder attending to some top windows and gradually moving down to the bottom. It was while I was at the bottom removing the putty from the remaining few frames that the pivot window above fell off its hinges and plummeted down. Of course, I was directly underneath but did not realise it had fallen until I stood up and knocked against it. There it was hanging by the rope that was used to open it, and it was swinging no more than six inches above where my head had been. It took me a long while for me to realise how lucky I had been, especially as it must have weighed at least a hundredweight. It could have killed me. After that incident I became more safety conscious and realised that the building trade could be dangerous if you were not careful.

Now I was earning regular money my thoughts began to focus on a possible holiday. I really needed one as my last was when I was still at school and that was a few years ago. I did not have any close friends that I could go with and I was too old to go with Mum and Tom, so my thoughts turned to Sister Sue. Sue's marriage had failed (not too surprising), so she was back on her own again. Mum suggested that I get in contact with her and discuss a holiday. I spoke to her promptly and we both agreed that a break would do us good. Sue's job at the bank was the main problem but she soon phoned back to me to say she had fixed a week in June, so all that was left was for me to get the same week off work. It was not a problem and after discussing where we would be going, we decide to hire a caravan for a week in Devon.

Back at work, with the holiday booked the time seemed to go a lot slower. My 21st birthday was celebrated in May and the holiday seemed to loom larger on the horizon. Eventually the date came round and Sue travelled down from Norfolk, and early the Saturday morning we jumped in my car and set off.

It was a very arduous journey for me, not just because of the traffic but something much more troubling. Early on during the drive I began to get a lot of anxiety. I started to feel that I would lose control of the car and have an accident. However much I tried to tell myself I was being stupid, it did not help. All the way along the motorway the feelings persisted, so I had to keep my speed down and stay as much as possible in the inside lane, even then my anxiety would not relent. We reached the end of the motorway, with Sue unaware of what I was feeling. I felt relieved we were on a normal road once more but this turned out to be premature as I now became almost petrified that I would steer into the oncoming traffic. By the time we reached our destination I was mentally exhausted. I had not been able to relax at all and all I wanted to do was flop down and rest.
I tried to forget the day's troubles and concentrate on the holiday. I could not understand why I should have had the anxiety and hoped it was just a one off situation. We went out for a drink that evening and I had several. I was of the opinion that I deserved a drink and made the most of the opportunity.

    We toured around Devon for the major part of the holiday visiting most of the big coastal resorts. As the week went by I began to feel more and more unhappy, although I tried not to show it. I was as usual eager for love and so far had not had a sniff of it. The main problem with going on holiday with your sister is that everyone thinks you are a couple, so I made the point of revealing the truth at every opportunity.

    Things took a change for the better on the

Wednesday of the week, when we visited Paignton. We managed to park the car near the sea front and went exploring in the town. We visited the pier and came across the resident fortune teller which proved to hold an attraction for my sister. As we stood outside we entered into a discussion and it was agreed that Sue would like a reading, so we went in and found she could have one immediately.

I waited outside and started to think about having a reading myself, although I was not prepared to pay the full amount. I must have waited a good half an hour before Sue emerged from the room, and by the look on her face she was pleased with what she had heard. She confirmed this and urged me to go in myself. Picking up courage I went in and told the lady I could not afford a full reading so she offered me a reduced session at a lower cost, which I accepted. Initially, I was full of trepidation but very quickly lost that feeling as I listened to her words. The first thing she said was that although I was on holiday I was feeling miserable. She then went on to say that I would meet a girl within two days and have a relationship with her. She related a few other things to me and finished up by saying that I would eventually settle down with somebody, but that was a long time in the future. I thanked her for the reading and departed to join Sue outside.

We swapped stories on our way back to the caravan and made light-hearted comments about them. I did not really believe that anything I had been told would come true, and would in fact go out of my way to prove what a load of rubbish it was. Sue commented that she would only have to wait until Friday to find out and I agreed with her.

We remained in Sidmouth for the rest of the

holiday relaxing and generally taking things easy. Friday came and we did the same that day, nothing eventful happened and by the evening the main topic of conversation was packing up and going home. We decided to go out for a final drink, but restricted ourselves to the local area, so we picked a pub that was close to the caravan. We sat and talked most of the evening and remarked that the lady on Paignton Pier had got it wrong because as time had past and nothing out of the ordinary had happened.

The pub was not very busy and the bar staff had time to talk, so it was little surprise when a barmaid who we had spoken to earlier came over and started to chat. She was very friendly, as well as attractive, and soon we were laughing and joking together. It was not long before I noticed that she was addressing more and more of the conversation to me at the expense of Sue, and it quite quickly became apparent that she fancied me. Her name was June and she was married but it did not seem to make any difference, because she seduced me and we ended up in bed. When morning came there was a smile on my face as big as a Cheshire Cat's.

Sue was not happy when we set off for home (she was feeling left out), but I soon talked her round. The conversation, once again, turned to the future and what the fortune teller had told us. It now had more meaning than before. We had both said our goodbyes to June and we all promised to write; I even got the hint that I might get a visit in Surrey in the not too distant future. So I left her with a kiss and a smile and thought of a possible reunion.

The journey home was better, but I was still troubled by a little of the anxiety I had felt the previous Saturday although it was not as bad.

Sue stayed in Surrey for the night and went back to Norfolk on the Sunday. Since her separation she was living in an old rectory somewhere out in the 'sticks' along with her cat and an elderly couple. I never asked her if she was happy, but I somehow knew she was not.

Life soon drifted back to normality after the holiday and there was still plenty of work to be done at Brookwood Hospital. I received regular letters from June and did a lot of thinking about her. The thoughts I had of her were soul-searching ones rather than love-struck ones. I tried to fathom out how I felt about her and whether there was any future for us, and decided it would be best to see her again. The opportunity arose very soon as Mum and Tom had arranged to go away for a weekend. Without hesitation, I wrote to June and asked her to come that weekend and within a few days I received a reply saying, 'Yes'. After that we made the necessary arrangements and I waited in anticipation for the weekend in question. It came and I met her at the station after work on the Friday evening. As soon as we arrived home we satisfied our lust for each other for a couple of hours, she was a lot more experienced than me so I learnt a few new things as well! It was one of the best weekends I have ever spent and apart from making love, I particularly liked having a girl on my arm. When we went out, it gave me a sense of pride and contentment.

Very soon into the weekend, I realised that June was not the woman for me and when we parted we half arranged that we would meet again soon, to be confirmed by letter but I never wrote to her so I never saw her again. She continued writing to Sue and the last I heard was that she had had a miscarriage. I sometimes felt like writing to her in times of loneliness but did not, it would not have been fair and besides she would have probably told me to get lost!

Work continued and I became more and more depressed with it. I was beginning to feel trapped in my way of life and did a bit of thinking about my future, without coming to any real conclusions. My social life still revolved around the Hospital Club and working at the pub.

Keith began to figure in my life much more and we often drank together at the club, and became good friends. He was a bit of a rogue and certainly liked a pint, as I did, so we were quite well matched. As we became friends I learnt that he had been banned from driving because of drink, but it did not seem to bother him because he still carried on drinking and driving. Knowing this I began to be aware of myself and a similar situation. I was drinking and driving nearly every night and sometimes I had been well over the limit, so it was only a matter of time before I was caught unless I did something about it. But amongst bigger issues I tended to push this knowledge to the back of my mind and not want to face it.

Keith had a new girl friend, her name was Linda and he often brought her up to the club, so I got to know her quite well. She was a short and dumpy woman in her thirties with a very appealing face and a bubbly personality. It was very easy to like her and she soon became a friend of mine also. I often played gooseberry to Keith and Linda, but nobody seemed to mind because we got on so well together. Being with them was great, it helped take my mind off things and I always looked forward to our meetings. I never realised at the time how much their friendship would mean to me, but fate was soon to take over events.

Drinking was an escape to me but it also had its risks. One night when I was driving home from the club a police car following me started flashing its blue light. I decided that an immediate reaction was needed as I had been drinking, so I pulled over. A policeman walked over to my car and asked me to get out, he explained that I had crossed a white line and asked me if I had been drinking? I replied that I had had a couple, so he produced a breathalyser bag and asked me to blow into it. To my surprise the test was negative, and the police departed leaving me with just a caution.

A few weeks later I did an extremely foolish thing. I had arranged to meet Keith at the club and have a big drinking session. We did not drink beer as we usually did but started immediately on shorts, to see who had the greater capacity!

As the evening wore on we became more and more pickled and by closing time we were in such a state that we were almost incapable of walking. Instead of leaving my car and getting home some other way I insisted that I was more than capable of driving, so I did.

I made it somehow along the main road but turned into my estate too soon and hit a lamppost. The next thing I remember was being in the local police station giving a urine sample to be analysed. When I eventually arrived home in the early hours Mum and Tom were waiting for me and they were not in the best of moods. I heard a few days later that my sample was positive and that I was to be prosecuted.

I was allowed to continue driving until my court case came up, but as I still liked a pint I either walked to the Hen and Chickens or curtailed my drinking and went up to the Social Club.

I continued working some evenings at the Nag's Head where I told the landlord about my pending court case. He surprisingly recommended a solicitor to me and said he would put in a good word for me. While I was waiting to hear when the case would be I began to think that they had forgotten about it, but in April I heard from the court that I was to appear in front of the Magistrates at the end of May.

April was a month that was to prove eventful for me. I was working at the hospital as usual when I started to feel attracted to a lady much older than myself. I had seen her many times walking around and I had decided that I wanted to get to know about her, so I started to make enquiries and found out her phone number at work.

After many hours of plucking up courage I called her. I explained who I was and told her that I wanted a date. Her reply was that she (Joy) was very flattered but she already had a boy friend, however she would see me around. Thinking that was that I put her to the back of my mind and got on with my work.

The following week I was working alone round the back of the boiler-house when Joy came up to me and kissed me. I was most surprised, but pleased, especially when she said that there was much more to come. Every day we met at the same time and every day became steamier until I thought I was going to lose control of myself. Things were about to come to an abrupt halt however because someone I was about to meet would have a very big impact on my life, so big in fact that I would forget all about Joy, at least for a while. It happened that following weekend. I went to the social club on the Friday evening and joined the usual crowd up near the bar when a very sexy looking girl walked up and ordered some drinks. She had lovely long black, curly hair and was slim with a very well-formed bum which she showed off in skin tight jeans.

She had a very big effect on me and without thinking about it I got up and stood next to her at the bar. We somehow got talking and I knew immediately that I was hooked, she had a very bubbly personality and when she smiled her nose used to crumple up cutely. She seemed to be much at ease with me and I found her very easy to talk to. After introducing myself and finding out that her name was Kate, she went on to say that it was the first time she had used the club for a long time. I remember making it very plain that I fancied her and offered to buy her a drink to which she replied that she would like one later.

She did have a drink with me later and agreed to let me drive her home which was only a mile up the road. When we arrived at her house she asked me in for a little while explaining that her mother would be there. I did not mind as I enjoyed being with her and was pleased at the invitation.

As I followed her into the house we were greeted by a very surprising and familiar face. Her mother was Joy. At first I felt a little embarrassed as I could not believe it, but after a few moments I relaxed a bit as Joy showed no inclination to mention our previous liaisons. Within a few days Kate became very important to me, she filled my thoughts and I was on cloud nine most of the time. I tried to play it cool but failed, so I just hoped she felt the same way. After a few dates we had the opportunity to make love, so we took it and ended up in bed together where I tried, unsuccessfully, to consummate my love for her. It was painful for her as she was still a virgin and however much I tried she tended to back off. It was disappointing for both of us, but we agreed to try again another time. Unfortunately that time never came!

One evening, while I was on my way home from the Nags Head, I caught sight of a couple walking arm in arm along the road. At first it did not register that one of the two was Kate, but as I got nearer I realised the terrible truth, it was Kate!

I can not describe my feelings at the time except to say that I was devastated. We had been together for less than a fortnight and already she was being unfaithful. I did not sleep well that night, I had a terrible feeling of emptiness and isolation and my mind just did not rest. I somehow got through the following day without eating a thing and smoking myself to death. Mum, I am sure realised what was up but was tactful in not saying anything. I confronted Kate that evening but I was on a loser from the beginning. My emotions erupted and I lost any control that I still had left. I ended up making a complete and utter fool of myself and lost Kate for good. I cursed myself for being so weak!

One pint followed another, so by the time the bar closed I was drunk. All rational thought had gone and feelings of self-control followed the same way. I drove home feeling wiped out, I turned up the stereo in my car and promptly started to let all my anger and frustration surface. I threw the car from one side of the road to the other, screaming my head off. It must have taken half an hour or more until complete exhaustion had taken over and an awareness of self-preservation returned.

I could not remember driving at least five miles from home but I had somehow managed to, without disaster, and without being stopped by the police again. I made it home and, with Mum and Tom already in bed, collapsed on my own and drifted into unconsciousness. The next few days were hard, very hard and I declined the opportunity to visit the social club for the fear of seeing Kate and anyway I was so miserable. Time does heal and after about a week of staying in evenings I ventured down to the Hen and Chickens and found that this helped my recuperation considerably.

The following week I felt able enough to continue work up the Nags Head, I had previously told the landlord I was ill, so the week I had off did not matter and things returned to normal. I had continued my day job right through the troubled times but kept a low profile as much as possible and consequently neither saw or heard anything of Kate or come to that of her mother, Joy.

It was two whole weeks before I entered the social club again, but when I did everyone seemed pleased to see me and welcomed my reappearance. I saw Joy soon after and she was, as expected, very cool towards me. She said that there was no way we could pick up where we had left off and I was to forget any ideas to the contrary. So I had ruined both relationships with my possessiveness and weakness. I began to hate myself! Keith and Linda were there for me and helped me push Kate to the back of my mind. I talked to them a lot about her at first, but as the days drifted by the pain grew less and I started to get on with my life.

A week after celebrating my 22nd birthday I appeared in court. I put on m suit and briefed my solicitor, who put in a few good words for me and I received a £100 fine and a two year ban. I immediately had to hand in my driving licence to the court. The impact of the verdict was instantaneous and I wondered how I would get on for the next two years.

I kept my day job because the foreman was good enough to pick me up every morning and I carried on working at the Nags head for a while longer. As for my social life, I spent some free evenings at the Hen and Chickens and the rest Keith and Linda picked me up and took me out, either to the social club or elsewhere.

On the whole I did pretty well, but I was restless and this made me feel unhappy (even more unhappy than usual), something was missing out of my life, and I put it down to love.

Linda had a mother, I had never met her but Linda told me all about her. Apparently she was a clairvoyant and was supposed to be a good one (according to Linda). Remembering my holiday in Devon I asked Linda if it was possible for her mother to give me a reading. She said she would and all I had to do was to give her a personal item which she would pass on to her mother. So I gave her the St Christopher I always wore.

I waited impatiently for news, but I did not have to wait too long as about three days later Linda presented me with my necklace accompanied by the reading, handwritten on two pieces of note paper. I read it through slowly, taking in every word and when I reached the end I went back to the beginning and read it through again. After I had finished I sat back and smiled, a very broad smile, I must have looked a bit funny because Keith and Linda could hardly keep a straight face. Linda commented that I must have liked the reading and I replied that it was very good, but the answer in truth was well understated, because I was delighted.

As I sat there I thought to myself that even if I had written it myself I could not have done a better job and I felt a sense of contentment which I had not felt for a long time.

Many feelings entered my mind, but they were all positive. I could not believe how a few words on paper could make so much difference, but they did and to this day I can remember the major points of what Linda's mother wrote. The first thing that comes to mind is that she saw a vivid picture of Oslo in Norway, she then went on to say that although I had gone through a bad pattern emotionally, it would all end when I met a petite person possibly with dyed hair and very small feet. I would meet that person within a few months and would hold a deep love for her which would be reciprocated. Of course she said other things but they were not as significant as these points I have mentioned, which were very important to me at that time.

Throughout the following days I thought about my future a lot and wondered where Oslo came into the equation, was that the key to everything? Was I going to meet that girl in Oslo? I became confused and impatient and my feelings of depression started to come through once more. I decided I had to do something positive. I had some money from selling my car, so after much thought I decided that I would go to Oslo and tempt fate. When I told Mum where I was going she said I was being silly as I had previously let her read what Linda's Mum had written. Nevertheless, once I had made up my mind I was determined so I started making preparations. I booked a week off with both jobs and purchased an Apex flight ticket, which meant I had to wait a month. I also acquired a book with a list of hotels in Oslo from which I chose one that I could afford and rang them up and reserved a room for a week.

Keith and Linda shared my excitement about Oslo and could not wait for me to come back and tell them all about it. I never let on to anyone that I was expecting to meet the girl of my dreams while I was over there, but I think a few who had read the reading suspected it.

As the day of departure approached the butterflies in my stomach worsened, but I had made up my mind that nothing was going to stop me going. Nothing did and before I knew it I was in the car on my way to Heathrow airport. On arrival I said my goodbyes to Mum and Tom and felt totally alone as they disappeared into the distance.

Flying was always a dislike of mine and the flight to Oslo changed nothing. Nevertheless I arrived in one piece and rather than have a lot of hassle finding my hotel I decided to get a taxi. The hotel was rather a dingy place, but was clean and comfortable and was situated in the centre of the city.

Immediately after a clean up I went out and explored. Remembering why I was there I thought the best strategy was to check out the location of all the decent bars and night-clubs in my area of the city. To my surprise the number of bars were few and far between, but the ones I visited were very busy and expensive. I found one spot which was a bit cheaper and decided that it would become my favourite place to visit. I had an opinion that it was better to get your face known in one place rather than stay a stranger in many. One thing that surprised me was the number of coloured people in Oslo and I found it quite amusing to hear them speaking Norwegian! As for being understood, most people spoke English very well and liked to practice it at every opportunity.

As I lay in bed the first night my thoughts turned to the 'Little Lady' I was destined to meet and decided that nothing else mattered but my search for her.

The following day I did some more exploring and found that there was very little to do in the daytime except perhaps going on a boat trip around the fjords. I did this in the afternoon, but apart from the wonderful views nothing worth mentioning happened.

As I disembarked from the boat I noticed a ferry moored at the quay so I went over and investigated. I found out that it carried people over to the peninsula called Bygdøy. I decided that I would go over the next morning.

That evening I went to the bar that I had located and stayed for a couple of hours. Many people spoke to me and were very pleasant when they found out that I was English. So by the end of my first day I was very optimistic for the following week.

Bygdøy was a beautiful place, it had lots of trees and there were many houses dotted in between. I remember thinking how romantic it would be to take my 'Little Lady' there. I also found out that many museums were located there. During the next couple of days I visited them all, making them a very interesting couple of days.

Halfway through the week I began to get a bit desperate. Although I was getting around I had not even had a sniff of romance yet alone met my 'Little Lady'. I had met a nice girl in the bar one evening but was reluctant to pursue her because she was quite tall and certainly did not have little feet!

Again, lying in my bed meditating I decided that if I was fated to meet the 'Little Lady' I would whatsoever I did. Why not ask the other girl out and leave everything to fate, if indeed I saw her again.

Two days before leaving Oslo I saw the girl again and she said that she would go out with me but, with so little time left our relationship did not have a chance to develop. So I left Oslo with mixed emotions, but I felt more than anything that I had wasted my time and my money!

One thing I did get from my trip was that I enjoyed adventure and I enjoyed travelling, and knew that I would travel again and soon!

As I slipped back into routine at home with the memory of my trip still fresh in my mind I continued to think about my 'Little Lady' and wondered where I would meet her. I kept looking at Linda's mother's reading and soon realised that she had been right about Oslo regardless of why. So why would she not be right about the rest!

Keith and Linda continued to be good friends and took me out regularly, most of the time just up to the social club but it did not matter because I was grateful for their continued help. I missed not having a car especially in the evening when I was working at the Nags head, so I had to either scrounge a lift or cycle. My time at the pub was coming to an end because I was finding it harder and harder to stay on good terms with the landlord.

Shortly before I left, his daughter came to stay for a few days and I quickly got to know what she was like! I was standing behind the bar taking to her father when I felt a hand on my leg moving towards my bum. Finding it hard to keep a straight face I moved away from her, only to find that she followed me and carried on groping me! I pushed her into the kitchen and told her to stop doing it, to which she replied that she would only if I came into the pub the following evening. I promised that I would.

I kept my promise and found her waiting for me as

soon as I entered. We sat down at a table and were joined by her strict father and his wife. As she was only 15 I felt disappointed but knew that I would have an interesting evening. Right from the word go she could not keep her hands off me, so I did the same with her. Nearly all night we groped each other in front of her father and his wife and they did not suspect a thing!

The night ended as it had begun with the landlord's daughter waving me goodbye and following her father upstairs. I never saw her again as the next day she went home to her mother's. A week later I stopped working at the Nags Head after a big bust-up with the landlord.

The next six months passed relatively quietly. The work contract at Brookwood Hospital was reaching its end and with it another stage in my life. By the end of the year and the decade I had not seen a hint of the 'Little lady', but I carried on hoping although I was starting to get a little disillusioned again. A sort of depression appeared to take root and this seemed to trigger off some nasty little fears. One particular one which caused me some distress was the fear of losing control of myself and hurting people, especially if I was handling tools or knives and particularly if the person was more vulnerable like babies and the elderly.

In spite of my problems I remained philosophical and stayed convinced that everything would sort itself out as soon as I got a settled, happy life with a lovely wife

Early in the new year of 1980 I came to another discussion and that was that I would go on another trip, probably to Europe and definitely longer than a week. I did not decide when but the very thought lifted my spirits for a while.

The hospital job finished but luckily for me the firm started another local contract so I was able to continue working for them, with the foreman still picking me up every morning. By this time I had learnt many and varied aspects of the building trade and was always pestering to be given the chance to do the more skilled tasks.

Keith and Linda remained good friends and as the time passed we visited the social club less and less. In fact, we tended to stay a lot more over in Linda's area (Weybridge) and I quite often stayed on Saturday night and made a weekend of it. Of course, by this time I had got to meet Linda's mother and had several more readings, but none ever matched up to the first which I always kept on my person!

May became a significant month, not only because I celebrated my 23rd birthday but secondly I was made redundant and also that resulted in me finalising my plans for my trip abroad. I decided to get an Inter Rail ticket which allowed me to travel on any European Rail Network at no further cost for a month; this I remember cost me about £90. I also joined the Youth Hostel Association so that I could get cheap accommodation almost wherever I went as long as I referred to a map and went to the places that had a hostel.

I had decided on a destination, I would be going to the south of France. When I arrived there I would look for work and stay as long as I could. I needed various 'bits and pieces', so I purchased a rucksack and a tent and anything else that a traveller might need. The one other very important thing I bought was a diary so I am able to give a more detailed account of my trip than I could have from memory.

It was raining the day in late June when I left, but I

did not leave alone, I had the company of Mum, Tom, Keith and Linda. They all came to Southampton to see me off.

As the boat left the harbour I went up on deck to wave goodbye, I felt very emotional as the four figures disappeared into the distance and realised only then that I was starting the biggest adventure of my life. I relaxed by visiting the bar and having a few beers before once again going up on deck to watch the sea.

It was an enjoyable crossing and the boat arrived mid-afternoon at Cherbourg where, after disembarking, I headed for the local railway station. I had already planned where to spend the night and had chosen AlenHon station as my destination. Without any major mishaps the train pulled into AlenHon station in the early evening. Unfortunately it was still raining so I decided to shelter from it for a while and try to find out where the Youth Hostel was situated. I found out that I had a three kilometre trek to the hostel, so as it was getting late and the rain was easing off, I started my hike. After walking for about 20 minutes I came across a young couple parked by the side of the road. I explained to them that I was English and asked where the Youth Hostel was. They seemed to understand my limited French and very kindly gave me a lift and dropped me right outside the building.

The accommodation was adequate but I did not sleep that well, however I did not let it affect me and the following morning over breakfast I planned the day ahead. I walked to the station only to find that I had to wait until the early afternoon to catch the train I wanted, so I went into the café that was adjacent to the station and sat at the bar and ordered a beer. I soon attracted an interest among the locals also at the bar and it was not long before one particular Frenchman attempted to hold a conversation with me.

As the morning wore on and the number of empty beer bottles in front of me increased a certain rapport between the Frenchman and I was established. It was not long after that he insisted on showing me round the local church, which although not my scene, I tried to be enthusiastic about so that I would not hurt his feelings. I even took a couple of photographs for good measure. The time of the train's arrival drew near so I thanked my new found friend and returned to the station. The train (not like in England) was on time, and as I looked for a seat I noticed many other travellers with rucksacks aboard. My destination this time was Valence, it took all afternoon and it was well into the evening again before I arrived. I found the Youth Hostel just in time and was grateful for the bed it offered. After a better night's sleep I met a French couple who spoke fairly good English and had breakfast with them at a local café.

Avignon was my next 'port of call', this time I was lucky with the train and reached my destination by lunch time. I had one last train to catch, and that was to Nice, but I had to wait two hours on Avignon station. Up until then I had felt pretty good in myself, but as I sat on a bench watching trains come and go I suddenly started to feel afraid that I was going to lose control of myself and jump in front of a train. This was very frightening and I soon found that I was reluctant to move an inch and gripped the bench very tightly whenever a train appeared.

When I boarded the Nice train I was in a state of shock and it took me a good hour to recover my composure. I did not know why I felt these fears but I prayed for help to conquer them and also prayed for guidance on my adventure.

As the train reached southern France the weather became hot and sunny and it raised my spirits. The line hugged the coast right from Marseilles to Nice and the scenery was spectacular.

Nice was a very busy place even at dusk when I arrived. It had two Youth Hostels, but I was too late to find them open so I had a couple of drinks and caught another train back to Antibes which had caught my fancy on the way.

It only took half an hour to reach Antibes but that was long enough to meet two other English lads called Nick and Ross. They were travelling around just like me and as we talked we all found out we had a lot in common. We reached a mutual decision about getting off the train in Antibes feeling that there must be camp sites around. We began our search with optimism only to find that it was far too late and it was getting dark.

As the sun went down we found ourselves in a place just outside Antibes called Biot, where we had been told there were camp sites. We gave up our search for the day because by now we were tired and hungry. We found a suitable field and set up camp for the night, hoping upon hope that we would not be told to move on.

The sun's heat woke me about seven o'clock in the morning and I found that Nick and Ross were already up and striking camp. Anxious not to be left behind I hurried and got dressed and packed my things. It struck me later that maybe they wanted to be by themselves, but when I asked they denied it. Our search for a permanent campsite continued, firstly in Biot and then back to Antibes. We did not have much luck and by lunch time we were all completely knackered!

We relaxed on the beach that afternoon and I

quietly prayed to myself that we would find a campsite soon. It was a pleasant afternoon which we spent eating, swimming and sleeping, but it soon passed and we resumed our search at tea time. We walked for about three miles and arrived at a place called Cagnes-sur-mer. We past an inviting café by the railway station and we all looked at one another and without hesitation went back and ordered some beer. We were there all evening and by about midnight we were well and truly pissed. It took all our efforts to stagger outside; all we wanted to do was sleep. Luckily there was a building site opposite and at Nick's suggestion we crashed out in a partly finished villa.

We did not sleep well, apart from the fact that it was not comfortable we were woken at six thirty in the morning by the workmen. We all agreed that it was of paramount importance to find a camp site as fatigue had taken over and we were wilting under the sun.

We decided to leave the rucksacks at the station and after a short debate Ross agreed to stay with them, which enabled Nick and me to investigate the local area at a much quicker pace. We did not have to go far, we found a camp site about two kilometres from the station and there was room for us. It also had showers!

That evening we were clean, had eaten and were very, very tired. Nevertheless we stayed up chatting, had some more beers and got talking to our German neighbour who was a girl called Sylvia and on holiday. Sylvia was very friendly and asked if she could accompany us on a trip to Monte Carlo the next day and we agreed that she could. After another long day I got to my feet and said 'goodnight' to the others and virtually fell into my tent and fell asleep immediately.

The four of us caught the train to Monte Carlo the

next morning and spent the day sightseeing and lazing on the beach. I became fascinated by the large boats in the Marina and as evening came the owners and their guests dined on the sterns in full view of passers-by. It certainly showed me how the other half lived. Where ever we went there were beautiful women and it made me depressed, envious of all the men that had them on their arm.

Later that evening we went to the casino and although we did not spend much we enjoyed ourselves and Nick even managed to win £30. By the time we finished drinking at a very reasonably priced café we realised that we had missed the last train, so we went and sat in an all night café until dawn.

Once again knackered, we caught the first train. Sylvia got off at Cagnes-sur-mer but we carried on to Cannes as there were a lot of employment agencies there. Before looking for work we tried to get some sleep on the beach, which by then was fairly crowded.
I tried to chat up a lovely blonde girl from Canada who seemed rather friendly. I eventually asked her out and arranged to meet her at a local café the following evening. On refection I did not really think she would turn up but remained optimistic.

Being a Saturday, all the work agencies were closed so we decided to come back on the Monday. We left Cannes and arrived back at the camp site by tea time. After a shower and something to eat I left the others and walked round the local marina. It was a very pleasant evening with a cool breeze and my thoughts turned again to my 'Little Lady'. By now I started to wonder if I would ever meet her and I realised how much I needed her to give me hope for the future.

The next day, Sunday, we all went to Nice and

stopped at an attractive café and had a good lunch, after which we went to the beach.

We arrived back at the camp site around tea time once again and I had a shower and a change of clothes ready for my trip to Cannes to meet the Canadian girl. I arrived in good time and sat and had a couple of beers, but she did not turn up. Deep down I knew that she would not turn up, but it all served to reinforce my already low self-confidence.

Nick, Ross and I returned to Cannes on the Monday and checked all the agencies for work, which proved fruitless. The only positive note we got from the day was meeting an English couple who knew a boat owner in Antibes who was looking for a crew. We immediately went there and asked around only to find that the boat had left the previous week.

By this time Nick and Ross had decided to move on elsewhere and knowing that I did not figure in their plans I said that I would be staying. All four of us spent their final day on the local beach which turned out profitable for me.

While sun-bathing an oriental looking chap came up to us and asked whether we wanted to buy an ice-cream. I light-heartedly said, 'No, but I would like a job!' Without hesitation he said I could have a job and I could start in a couple of days. Although it meant trudging up and down a beach all day I said I would do it. We celebrated that evening with lots of beer and wished each other good luck as Sylvia said that she was leaving soon as well.

The following morning Nick and Ross packed their belongings and said goodbye. It happened so quickly that they were gone before I realised, once again, I felt that terrible feeling of isolation but I was equally determined not to let it beat me!

I spent the rest of the day and evening with Sylvia on the beach and had a really good time until I spoilt it by trying to proposition her. I thought that I had a jolly good chance and was dismayed and frustrated when she refused. What was wrong with me! That is the question I asked myself when I went to bed. I felt like crying but refused to allow myself to do it. I woke up the next morning to find that Sylvia had already left.

Being alone once again did not bother me deep down; it was like a whole new adventure. It was puzzling to me as to why I should feel isolated and sick in my stomach every time I was left alone, especially as I relished the challenge. It was as though my subconscious feelings were out of control.

Nevertheless this time I had work to go to, so when the time came I collected my polystyrene shoulder box and loaded it up with ice and ice-cream. I set off on my patch of beach trying to persuade the holidaymakers to part with their money. It was hard work and I began to sweat freely, but I carried on regardless only to find that by the end of the day I had only sold three ice-creams and all the rest had melted!

The boss of the outfit was not exactly happy with my efforts, but to my surprise offered me a job which he thought would suit me better. The job in question would mean working in the evenings and involved selling donuts and pizza to the holidaymakers outside a holiday park near Biot.

That evening the boss picked me up and drove me to my spot, which was right next to a line of African traders selling their native products. I set up my stall and said goodbye to my boss who said he would return about 10 o'clock. To my delight the holidaymakers were practically all English and they seemed very pleased to see me. I sold out of everything within 2 hours, and with me getting 10 per cent of the takings I worked out that I had made 300 Francs which was roughly £30, I was well pleased! I had really landed on my feet, and I started dreaming of the things I could do for the rest of the summer with all that money.

    The next day I spent lazily on the beach and pondered about my situation. If I could continue to work and earn as much, I would be in a very healthy financial situation and even after the season's ending I could continue my travels, or even return home for a while. It was a happy day for me, which was becoming a rare event and I began to think that maybe now the tide of life was turning and I could look forward to meeting my 'Little Lady' very soon.

    The evening started well, I was selling my donuts and pizzas quickly and was again well pleased. I had sold at least half when a Frenchman pulled up in front of my stall in a big car. It was quite easy to understand what he was talking about because he was very angry. He apparently owned a café up the road and since I had arrived his takings had slumped! I decided to act dumb and just gestured with my arms to which he seemed to back down and got back into his car. He started his car and reversed down the road a little way, he then drove back towards me at speed and sent my stall crashing all over the place. All my produce and takings were sent flying and I had to jump out of the way.

    The mad Frenchman drove off down the road and I was left there bewildered and shaking. Many people came to my aid and picked up the money that was lying all over the place, but apart from thanking them I did nothing else being still in a state of utter bewilderment.

Five minutes had passed and the Frenchman returned with two Doberman dogs and a younger man. The dogs were on a lead and seemed to be for protection more than anything else, as their owner stayed a good distance away from me.

Within another 5 minutes the police arrived and started talking to the man and then wandered across to me and tried to ask me questions. Once again, although I understood a little I decided to make out that I did not speak French. After a little while I was taken to the police car and driven to Antibes police station.
I was left sitting in the police station for at least two hours and had to put up with a prisoner pestering me. He was locked in the cell next to me, a cell which was only about four feet high and the same wide. I ignored him. When a police officer returned he asked me in broken English where I was staying. I told him and very quickly found myself back in a police car heading towards the camp site. On arrival the police talked to the owner for quite a while, then came back to me and said that I must leave the camp site in the morning and immediately leave France!

I was devastated and could not believe what had happened over the last few hours. I did not have many options open to me. I could go further west along the coast and try to find another camp site and work or go home. I decided on the latter as all my sense of adventure had temporarily disappeared and besides all that, I had nearly run out of money. I was very disappointed that I had lost my stall at such a great pace and felt depressed at how things had worked out considering how euphoric I was the previous day. My boss was also disappointed but was not angry with me for what had happened.

My first real adventure was over and I felt low when I boarded a train, but at least I had had a few experiences that I could tell others about. I had to change trains to get to Paris, but I managed to get a seat when it mattered and spent the time thinking of what might have been. While I was half asleep I thought that I felt my knee being rubbed and looked up and saw a girl sitting opposite me move her foot. This seemed to happen a couple more times throughout the journey so when she got up to go to the toilet I followed her and waited outside rather exited, thinking I might at last have a sexual liaison! But alas, again it was not to be because she came out, completely ignored me and returned to her seat.

    I caught another train form Paris to Calais and then a ferry to Dover arriving home eventually at four thirty the following day, completely knackered!

I'M SURE I'LL WAKE UP IN A MINUTE!

Life was not easy on my return from France. I was not very happy; in fact I was downright depressed. I tried to lift myself, thinking of various reasons why I should feel like I did. The answers I came up with were: that I did not have a job; I did not know what I wanted to do as regards a career; I did not have transport (because of my ban); and most important of all, I did not have a girl friend. Things never felt this bad before and I was starting to feel desperate. I knew I had to do something and fast!

In my desperation I turned to God and did a lot of praying, but even that tended to have little effect on me but I continued doing it. I started to dwell on the past and looked at all my failures, and then started to blame myself for my inadequacies coming to the conclusion that I was a prat and could not do anything right! I was ashamed of myself.

All through this period I suffered from chronic heartburn and bought various remedies to control it. Mum was sympathetic and said I was worrying too much. I think she sensed that I was not very happy, but I always snapped at her if she said anything.

In desperation I bought a book about working abroad and decided that I would like to go grape picking in France during September, so I wrote away and booked my place on the coach and handed over the relevant amount of money. I worked out that I had just enough cash put by for spending money on the trip and would have to live off my dole money until the time came to leave.

The desperation lifted a little and I saw this as a sign that I had made the right decision and that everything would work out once I went on the planned trip. Once again my 'Little Lady' came into my head and I started dreaming about her and the experiences I would go through on my trip.

My biggest enemy was time. I still had about six weeks to kill and they came to feel more like six months. Keith and Linda remained good friends and took me out regularly. I also went up to the pub when I could afford it.

The days trickled past and the depression returned, even my constant thoughts of France did not seem to shift it. I prayed for strength to see me through the remaining weeks. I still believed that my next trip would be the making of me and everything would work out, if I could just hang on a little while longer.

September arrived and I learnt that the harvest was late and I would not be leaving until October. So, I had to endure another three weeks! I built up a resolve in me that whatever I had to go through before October I would conquer it and nothing would stop me living my dream.

Nothing did, although it was hard I made it, and on the 9th of October 1980 I said farewell to my family and friends and once again caught the train for London where I was to join the coach for France.

By the time I arrived in London I was feeling low. I should have felt excited but for whatever reason I was full of apprehension. I met Dad and we went for a couple of drinks. It was good to see him as it had been a long time since our last meeting. I had cheered up a little when I said my goodbyes to Dad and joined the coach at Victoria.

The coach journey to Southampton was not the best trip I've had. It took all my resources to stop myself from jumping up and running off the vehicle, but somehow I made it and on arrival I visited the toilets and was violently sick! I used the toilets twice, and the second time I remember being laughed at by some young boys who thought it was extremely funny that I should be throwing up! I felt like going home, but resisted and somehow knew that if I went home I would have bigger problems than I already had.

On board the ferry I started talking to a younger chap whose name was Graham and subsequently found out that he was going to the same chateau as me. I started to calm down a bit but still felt apprehensive. I decided that I had to try anything to take my mind off things. I suffered all through the night and consequently had very little sleep and by the time the ferry docked at Le Havre I was a mental wreck.

It took the coach all the next day to reach Bordeaux, luckily I sat next to Graham and that helped a lot. The first chateau to find was for six, three girls and three men including myself and Graham, but the organiser had a lot of trouble finding it. As the evening wore on a lot of people started to get annoyed, including me, and I made it known more than anyone else. I really gave the organiser a bad time and realised after a short time that this annoyance seemed to solve my sickness and from then on I just felt so exhausted that I fell asleep.

When we finally arrived at the chateau the six of us were introduced to the proprietor, who was a nice man, but he spoke very little English so it was left to his wife to translate.

We were shown our sleeping quarters that were pretty basic with six bunks and an open hearth, but there was one luxury and that was a shower that actually worked! The six of us were to share the same room, which was a bonus because I had already had my eyes on one of the girls.

The rest of the day was spent getting to know each other and sitting down to lunch and evening meals. The food was good, but unfortunately for me it had garlic in it (I hate garlic) so I only ate a little and washed it down with lashings of the red wine that was on offer.

That night the third guy who shared our room decided to light a fire and sat up talking to one of the girls until two o'clock in the morning. So, with the heat from the fire and the noise of their talking, I got to sleep very late.

In the early hours I dreamt about something horrific and consciously jumped out of bed to avoid whatever was about to happen in my dreams, and as I was on the top bunk I was lucky I did not hurt myself.

The next day we were put to work and because I was fairly broad I was given the task of porter. This involved walking up and down the rows with a big container on my back while the pickers tipped their grapes in it.

I was pleased with the task of porter because our pickers soon suffered from bad backs. We were the only English people employed at the chateau, the rest were Spanish.

That night I decided that four out of the six of us were getting along fine, but I realised after consultation with the other three that the remaining two would have to be spoken to. They were always the first to grab the food at meal times and often took more than their fair share. They had already upset me with their antics of the previous evening and if they did the same again I would definitely have to say or do something about their selfishness.

My quickly gained reputation from the coach came into play that night as once again the fire was lit and the talking started. I made myself very plain, abrupt and to the point, telling the two offenders to go outside if they wanted to talk and also that I would pour water on the fire if they continued to be selfish especially at mealtimes. They shut up at once!

The same thing happened to me in the early hours as the previous evening. I dreamt again and found myself jumping out of bed, only this time I hurt an ankle, but luckily not too badly that I could not work. On subsequent nights I swapped bunks with Graham and the annoying thing was that I never leapt out of bed again!

After a few days Graham and I struck up a friendship with the proprietor's son and very so started having nights out with him and his mate. Graham spoke better French than I but I was picking it up fast so between us we did pretty well at making ourselves understood. For once I started to enjoy myself; there was no return to the previous problem except for slight depression that I learned to live with.

My only other real problem was communicating with the females I came into contact with and that were as big a frustration as ever.

The major frustration was with the girl I fancied in our room. She knew I fancied her but as usual I did not know how to break the ice. However, one evening an opportunity presented itself. It was after supper and we all decided to stay in the dining room and drink wine. As the evening wore on we showed signs of being worse for wear and I turned my attention to the girl in question. We had a chat, and the conversation started off cleanly but soon changed to the subject of sex and relationships. I made sure that I left her in no doubt what I would like to have done with her.

After a short while she abruptly got up and left

saying she was going to bed. I took this action of hers as a statement that she did not want to know me, so once again thinking I had been rebuffed I carried on drinking with the others. About an hour later we decided to go to bed, so we emptied our glasses and staggered back to our room.

The light was on in the room and surprisingly the object of my desire was lying on my bunk reading. Now I was rather drunk and feeling sorry for myself. Still thinking that she did not want to know me I asked her to move so that I could go to bed. She did as I asked, but come the morning she more or less ignored me and I eventually managed to realise the reason why. Once again I had an opportunity and once again I missed it. I was very, very, annoyed with myself and almost tore my hair out with frustration because I knew I would not get a second chance.

It took a few days to forget my foolishness, it would have been nice to escape to a pub and get drunk but unfortunately there were none in the area. I had to be content with drinking the rough wine they provided at the chateau, and that was beginning to taste like vinegar! Our stay at the vineyard lasted just over a fortnight and to celebrate the end of the harvest the proprietor and his wife laid on a party. They brought out last year's bottled wine for all the workers, and joined in the celebrations themselves, but after about two hours everyone had had their fill of wine and departed to spend their last night in the sleeping accommodation that had been provided for the duration.

Much discussion went on by us 'Brits' as what to do next. We had been told that picking was still going on in central France, so that was one option. The other was to return home. The latter was out of the question as far as I was concerned, so, after talking to Graham and persuading him that as it was on the way home, we could hitchhike north and find more work. The others decided to head for home by train.

The next day we all wished each other luck and said goodbye, and headed off in different directions. It had been a good experience in many ways and although everyone had been tired with aching backs most of the time, we still had had a few laughs.

Graham and I had decided to head for Chinon, as it was in central France and had a Youth Hostel. It took us half the day to walk to the other side of Bordeaux and find the right road, but after that we got our first lift fairly quickly. It was the first time either of us had hitchhiked and I, for one, found it exciting. I loved the uncertainty of it and revelled in the feeling of freedom it gave, every lift was different and every destination new.

We arrived in Chalon early in the evening and found the hostel quite easily although we were lucky to find it still had a few beds available. It was not hard to learn where the work was as everybody in the hostel was looking. There was a special bus that called at the hostel every day to collect people and take them to different chateaux. We retired early to make sure we were not left behind in the morning.

The work proved to be demanding as I was picking the grapes this time and I soon decided that the agony (from my back) was too much to bear for another day, so I quickly had a change of plan and decided to head for the French Alps to try and catch the early skiing season. I had a chat with Graham, who was also complaining about his back, and found that he'd had enough of the rough life and was returning to England in the morning. By now it was the end of October and after various enquiries I found out that the winter season did not start until December, so my ultimate plans had to be put on hold for the time being. Instead I thought about continuing my journey through France and possibly into Germany and even Switzerland. There was no rush, but I had to be careful or otherwise I would run out of money and be forced to return home.

Returning home was the last thing I wanted to do. I knew there was nothing there for me and besides I was even starting to enjoy myself, something I had not done for a long time if ever. The key to my enjoyment seemed to be the travelling, so I promised myself that I would not stay long in the same place, except of course, until I found my destiny. I felt confident I would know when it happened.

With Graham gone home I decided to head east for a while so I elected to go to the Alsace region of France. One of the most important things in my possession at that time was my map of all the Youth Hostels in Europe and, after consulting this, I chose Strasbourg as my destination. It was not that far (only about 200 miles) and I thought I could easily make it in one day.
My journey that day was a good one and gave me plenty of time to locate the hostel. Hitchhiking in that part of France seemed easier, so my spirits were high and as I lay in bed that night I started to think that I could go anywhere in Europe without much trouble at all. Unfortunately, I was soon to find out that that was strictly not true.

While relaxing at the Youth Hostel I got talking to another English guy called Andy. He was hoping to get a job in France so he could improve his French, but was uncertain of his plans. After talking to him and consulting various maps we came to an agreement that

Chamonix in the French Alps was a good destination. We studied the best route to take and agreed that we should do the journey together, aiming to go our separate ways after Chamonix.

As there was no real hurry we decided to go to Mulhouse the next day. Mulhouse is situated on the French-Swiss border and as we intended to visit Switzerland, it was an ideal place to start from.

The next day we said farewell to Strasbourg and leisurely made our way out of the city in the direction of Mulhouse. We arrived by lunch time after getting a lift from a farmer, sitting amongst the straw in his pickup truck. It was a lovely town and as it was virtually on the borders of three countries (France, Germany and Switzerland) it had a very mixed culture. It was such an interesting place that Andy and I made up our minds to stay for a couple of nights. The Youth Hostel was well located in the town and had a similar character to the rest of the town's architecture.

We spent an enjoyable day in Mulhouse, but by the end of the second evening I started to get itchy feet again and was eager to move on. That night we planned our next move and chose to head into Switzerland and take a look at Zurich. The border was only about 25 miles so it was not an ambitious task, but we were soon to find out that hitchhiking in Switzerland was not at all easy.

We crossed the border without much fuss and walked into Basel. It did not take us long to locate the road to Zurich and found what we thought to be an ideal spot at which to thumb a lift. We were there for five hours and by the time we managed to get a ride it was the middle of the afternoon, so we arrived in Zurich in the early evening. By the time we had fed ourselves we only had an hour to find the local Youth Hostel. We did not find it!

We wandered around the city looking for suitable places to sleep as there was no way either of us wanted to spend money on a hotel. Our search finally took us to the railway station and there we noticed various goods wagons further along the track. Being careful not to be seen we made our way along the rails and reaching the wagons proceeded to look for an open one in which we could get our heads down. We found one, and again being careful we climbed aboard and inspected our sleeping quarters.

It was dry and fairly clean inside the wagon, so we decided it was as good as anywhere else to sleep. Once we had rolled out our sleeping bags and removed our footwear we closed the doors only to find it was virtually pitch black, so I opened the door a little bit to let some light in.

We slept surprisingly well, but woke early to find a lot of activity going on outside. I suggested to Andy that it might be a good idea to get up and vacate the wagon just in case we found ourselves in Eastern Europe. We packed our rucksacks quickly but in my haste I left behind my seaman's knife that I had acquired in my navy days, so I was a little bit annoyed.

It was a cold morning and we searched for a café where we could get breakfast and clean up. As we sat eating our meal we discussed our next move. We both agreed that hitchhiking in Switzerland was a dead loss, and as we were heading for the French Alps it was not practical either. The only other alternative was the train. As we were both eager to get to Chamonix we decided that it was worth the money and when breakfast was finished we headed back to the railway station.

After checking the route we found we would have to change trains at Geneva, but that was not a real problem as Chamonix was very near to it and besides if we wanted to stay in Geneva a short while we could and it also had a Youth Hostel. The fare was very reasonable as well, and I remember thinking that it was the only thing in Switzerland that was cheap!

Once on the train Andy and I decided to try to sleep, but our minds were soon changed when we saw the scenery out of the window. Never in my life had I seen such beautiful countryside, even in my days in Scotland could not compare, it was magnificent. All the way through the three hour journey I did nothing but admire the mountains and valleys, lakes and rivers and the chalets that were so typical of Switzerland. I wished upon wish that I had a 'Little Lady' with me to share such beauty.

We arrived in Geneva too soon for my liking and as it was only lunch time decided to explore the city. It was well worth seeing, but after a couple of hours Andy and I agreed to carry on our journey to Chamonix. Another spectacular train journey ensued. At some points the train climbed at an angle of 45 degrees and I wondered how it was able to do it. Once again, as we climbed, the scenery was wonderful and it dawned on me what new adventure I might face at the end of the line.

There was no snow in Chamonix when we arrived, so we were a little disappointed but on reflection we knew it was a tall order especially when it was only the beginning of November. We found the Youth Hostel without any problems and asked the Warden if it would be possible to stay for a few weeks if necessary and in broken English he replied, 'Yes, it would be possible'.

A couple more English lads were staying at the hostel and we quickly became acquainted. They too were looking for work and after a week had found nothing and you could tell that they were becoming very disillusioned. After further conversation they told us about where you could advertise for work and which newspaper to buy but warned us that we were a month too early, especially for the skiing season.

As the days came and went, Andy and I became familiar with every inch of Chamonix but also realised that the other two English lads (who had now moved on) were right. There was no snow in Chamonix and while that continued there were no skiers, which meant no seasonal work. We were very disappointed and on the fifth day after our arrival we had a conference about what to do next. Andy was very keen to stay in France and find work. So was I, but Andy wanted to go back to Mulhouse for a few weeks. I was aware that my money was running out and wanted to return to the south of France, where I had heard there was nut picking going on. We decided to see the weekend out in Chamonix and in the meantime think about our options.

Fate however took a hand and the very next morning the Warden of the Youth Hostel turned nasty and demanded that we leave immediately. Both Andy and I were very angry with his attitude because we had always been clean and tidy, and quiet. He was adamant though and we had to pack up and leave.

As we were on the train going back to Geneva, Andy told me that he was going back to Mulhouse whereas I planned to go to Lyons and see what information I could pick up about seasonal work in the area. We parted with a hand shake and wished each other good luck, and went our separate ways. Looking back at our relationship I realised that we never really became friends, but were glad of each other's company for a little while.

With the dream of working in the mountains gone, at least put on hold, I became aware of the need for another goal otherwise I knew I would become depressed again. My initial goal was to get to Lyons and find the Youth Hostel so I could plan in relative comfort. With this in mind I walked across the border back into France and started to hitchhike once again.

I had a successful day and covered the short distance in no time at all, arriving in Lyons in the middle of the afternoon. It took me a while to find one of the two Youth Hostels in the city, but by the early evening I was lying in my bunk pondering the future. I had already asked about the work situation in the area but had drawn a blank, so I needed to think of something and quickly! While I was thinking my mind began to wander and I started to dream about a certain 'Little Lady' and all the things we could do together and how happy I would be. At one point I was so emotional about it that tears filled my eyes and started to roll down my cheeks. It was then that I started to realise that the most important thing to me was to have a relationship and that nothing else really mattered. Ever since I came back from Oslo I had not really tempted fate, so maybe now was the time to start once again and look for the 'Little Lady' whom I had dreamt about for so long.

As I lay on my bunk I began to think about Scandinavia once more and started to imagine that I was fated to go there again. If that was the case then I thought, well, why not go there tomorrow! This thought started to excite me and I saw this excitement as a sign that at last I had discovered my destiny. I would hitchhike to Denmark. After all it was in 'The Common Market' so I could still be employed there, but most of all it was full of Scandinavian girls! Where better to go than the capital, Copenhagen?

I did not sleep very well that night as I was so excited and could not wait for morning to start the journey to my destiny, find the love of my life, and at last find happiness. Nothing was going to stop me, even if I had to walk there I would. I was going to Copenhagen and that was it as far as I was concerned. The weather when I started must have been in the high sixties and like the weather I was optimistic. I got a lift north almost immediately and believe it or not ended up back in Chalon, but this time I was not interested in staying there. I wanted to carry on with my journey hoping to reach the German border by the evening. My hopes were dashed as I waited for another lift, it took at least four hours before a lorry pulled up beside me and offered a lift. Looking back though it was a good lift because the driver was very friendly and bought me a meal as well as helping to improve my French. When he dropped me off near the border I thanked him whole heartedly and assured him that I could afford a place to stay for the night. In reality I did not have a place to stay and as it was very late I decided to find a field where I could sleep for the night.

After a fitful night's sleep I was on the road very early and started looking for a café where I could eat a hearty breakfast. I found one more or less on the French-German border and used the rest of my French currency on a meal. It was worth it because I felt a lot better with a full stomach and was then ready to continue my journey.

Crossing the border was a doddle, I was just

waved on, and there were not any customs! My previous lift had done me proud because the driver had assured me that there was a motorway (autobahn) near the border and he was right. I only had to walk about two miles before I found it and as a bonus there was a junction right there!

There were other people thumbing a lift when I got into position, but I need not have worried because cars seemed to be stopping all the time. I had been there about a quarter of an hour when I was approached by a young lad around 16. He seemed upset and told me in broken English that a male motorist was hassling him and would it be all right if he stood with me! I agreed, as I felt sorry for him, so the two of us thumbed a lift together. It was not long before a car stopped beside us and the driver, a pretty young lady, said we could have a lift as far as Hanover. So we got in.

Hanover was over half the distance through Germany so I was well pleased and it was even better having such a lovely travelling companion. About 20 miles up the road we said goodbye to the young lad. He thanked us and wished me good luck on my journey, then waved as we continued on.

My driver was about my age and very attractive with shoulder length blonde hair. She was very friendly and it was not long before I felt attracted to her and started to enjoy the journey very much. As we covered the miles the conversation became more relaxed and intimate. She started to talk about her boy friend and how she had left him in Strasbourg while she came home on leave. She also told me that she worked for the Common Market as an interpreter and that she had met many nationalities, but preferred the English and especially English men!

Until then our conversation was very easy and friendly, but as usual I messed a very promising relationship up. The trouble started when she asked me if I was going to Denmark because of the lovely girls. Without thinking I replied that I intended to meet my future wife and settle down. To that answer she went very quiet and we hardly spoke for the rest of the journey. This gave me time to think and realise what I had said. When it dawned on me I could have curled up into a little ball. Once again I had ruined a potential intimate relationship by being too intense and putting myself across like a wet blanket, which I was!

As we approached Hanover it was the middle of the afternoon and I was getting very hungry again. We pulled into a motorway service station and I asked my 'friend' if she would join me, but she declined and said goodbye. I gave her my thanks and watched her disappear into the distance leaving me thinking what might have been.

Another disaster! I did not have any German money; all I had was travellers' cheques. I enquired at the cafeteria but they could not change them, I was stuck! I had two alternatives. I could go in to Hanover to a bank or I could continue my journey and change some money on the ferry across to Denmark.

After some thought, I chose to carry on my journey even though I had roughly 100 miles to go. So trying to forget about hunger I once again started to hitchhike. It took about an hour to get another lift, but it was a bad one. The driver of the car that stopped misunderstood me and had to drop me off at the next service station. It was getting dark by then and what's more, it started to snow!

Committed to my journey, I carried on determined

not to get down hearted. There were still a lot of vehicles on the road and my determination paid off, another car pulled up. The driver seemed a nice man and spoke pretty good English. I told him about my final destination and he said there was a service area just outside Hamburg where a lot of lorry drivers stopped for the night and that many of them were heading for Denmark. I thanked him for the information and asked him to drop me there.

By the time we arrived it was 10 o'clock and it was still snowing, but I was in good spirits. I said goodbye to my lift and looked around at all the lorries parked there and noticed that most of them had their curtains drawn, which meant that the drivers were asleep. I found a lorry that had Copenhagen on it and resigned myself to a sleepless night while I waited for the driver to wake up.

It was a long night. The snow continued falling and I had no real shelter from it. The worst part of the wait was the hunger, it had been nearly 24 hours since I had eaten and my mouth tasted foul. Every now and then I ate a little snow, but the combination of that and cigarettes brought on heartburn from which I could get no relief. By the time the sun rose I felt like a zombie. My spirits were high though and I remember thinking that I would not have changed a thing, I was experiencing life and somehow I thought it would all end in happiness!

It was seven o'clock when my lorry driver awoke and, with my long wait apparently over, I went across to him and asked whether he was going to Copenhagen. He said he was but that he did not give lifts. I was flabbergasted and tried to tell him that I had waited all night for him, but he was unmoved and suggested that I should try some of the other drivers.

Leaving him to it I looked around to see who else I could ask and by chance the lorry driver next to me was just waking up. I tapped on his window, which he opened and I asked him where he was going and to my astonishment he answered in a distinctive Scottish accent! He told me he was going to Sweden and that meant he was travelling through Denmark to get there. He said I could have a lift to Copenhagen and would I like to join him for breakfast? I thanked him and added that I did not have any German money, but said that I would pay him back on the ferry. I do not think food has ever tasted so good and I made a complete pig of myself. My new mate commented on my appetite and I told him how long it had been since I had my last meal. He laughed!

It was warm in the cab of the lorry, and a combination of that and the big meal was enough to send me to sleep. I would have slept but the driver wanted to talk, so every time my eyes closed he would purposely start another conversation.

We arrived at the ferry in good time. My driver went to the booking office and told them I worked for his company and returned with the news that I did not have to pay for the crossing. Once aboard I changed some travellers' cheques and obtained some Danish money after which I went back to my driver who was sitting in the lounge. Sitting nearby was the other driver who had refused to give me a lift and when I saw him I put up my hand, but he did not acknowledge me.
The crossing to Denmark went smoothly and only took a couple of hours, so we were soon back on the road again. I started to get a little excited as we approached Copenhagen and began to wonder what further

adventures were waiting for me. The first thing to do when I arrived was to find the Youth Hostel so I could hopefully have a base to work from while looking for work. I had to find work and fast because my supply of money was running out.

I was dropped off on the outskirts of the city, so I had a bit of walking to do. It did not bother me, however, as the realisation of how far I had come in such a short time dawned on me. I began to feel really tired again as I walked and was looking forward to getting my head down.

It took almost two hours to find the Youth Hostel, which was a modern building on the outskirts of the city centre. I was well and truly knackered as I finally fell into bed around eight o'clock that evening. I had not even bothered to eat before turning in, nor did I try to familiarise myself with the surroundings, but I had my own room and that was a bonus.

I slept round the clock and as I lay in bed early in the morning, I began to think about the situation I was in and to make plans. The most urgent need was money, as I only had enough to last a week and did not have any to get back to England with. I realised that it was the first time I had thought of returning home since I had left and it bothered me. My real goal was to make my future in Denmark and to find my partner, that wonderful 'Little Lady' that had so far proved to be elusive. I said a small prayer as I lay there, asking for the happiness I had sought for so long.

The day proved to be fruitless. I went round every work agency in Copenhagen without any joy and arrived back at the hostel tired and depressed. Yes, the depression had returned with a vengeance and with it went my optimism and hope for the future. As I lay on my bed tears began to fill my eyes and right at that moment I felt like the loneliest person in the world! I went to bed that night hoping that I would not wake up, but of course I did.

The following morning I decided to go round the agencies again, and if I did not find any work or at least some hope of work I would pack up and go home. After lunch I approached a shop that attracted my interest. It looked like a book shop, but on closer examination only one book was displayed, 'Dianetics' by Ron L. Hubbard. As I stood there I noticed a sign that asked if you were depressed and offered help. Feeling I had nothing to lose I entered the shop to investigate and was immediately approached. The man was at a guess about 45 and had a big bushy beard. He greeted me with a smile but made me feel apprehensive because he had very piercing eyes. In spite of this I filled out a questionnaire that he gave me, which asked about things, people and situations that tended to make me depressed. When I had finished the man read my answers and commented that he could help me get over my depression and led me into a room at the back of the shop.

As I waited, I began to think that maybe my prayers had been answered and at last I was on the right track. The man returned and told me that his organisation was called 'The Church of Scientology', and that if I became a member I would certainly become less depressed and more confident. He then introduced me to another lad about my age and said he would look after me for the rest of the day.

The lad, whose name was Erick, was very friendly and asked me if I wanted to have supper round his parents that evening,. I said I would be glad to and he

was very pleased. While I waited in the shop I got talking to an Australian who, like me, had become interested the same day. As we talked he told me that they said they would get him accommodation and a job if he joined the 'Church'. We both agreed that we did not care a toss about the 'Church', but liked the idea about the accommodation and work. When Erick returned I promised to keep in touch with the 'Aussie' and as I left we both exchanged knowing looks.
Erick's parents were nice people and seemed to support him, but I gained the impression that it was through loyalty more than anything else. As the evening wore on I became more and more uncomfortable in Erick's company, he seemed to be obsessed with the 'Church' and had the same overbearing attitude as the bearded man in the shop.

After a couple of hours praising the 'Church', Erick produced a contract and gave it to me to read. It more or less stated that anyone who signed it would put the 'Church' before anything else and would use any spare time doing work for the cause. By now I was convinced I was getting involved in a cult and into dangerous territory, however, I needed work and a place to live so I signed the contract, which, incidentally was for five years.

Within two days I was offered a flat that was situated about 10 miles outside Copenhagen. I took it, but used nearly all the rest of my cash up by paying the deposit. What was worse was that I had to commute by train every day that sapped my resources even further. Meanwhile, I played along with the 'Church' in the hope of being offered paid work, but none was forthcoming and I was forced by circumstances to write to Mum and ask her to send me a hundred pounds.

I met a lot of hostility while doing 'Church' work, work which involved giving out leaflets and general office duties. I was also encouraged to attend classes, where I was educated in Scientology and its founder, Ron L. Hubbard!

With no work in sight I decided to sever my links with the 'Church' and remained in my flat awaiting the money from England. I was being forced to make a decision about my future and began to feel that I had no option but to return home and try to make a life for myself there.

With the decision made I became despondent and depressed again, but I knew I had made the right choice, so when the money came I made my plans. I would get a train to Esbjerg and then catch the ferry from there.

The day of my departure came, so with my rucksack packed I vacated the flat and set off for Copenhagen railway station. While I was waiting for the train for Esbjerg I ran into my Australian friend, but he was far from pleased to see me! Apparently half the 'Church' members were looking for me and I was to report to them immediately. Of course, I told the Aussie that that was impossible and asked him why he was so serious. His answer knocked me for six. He told me that he was now heavily involved in the 'Church' and wanted to stay with them indefinitely and he would report my whereabouts to the other members.

I was very relieved when my train left the station with me on board and it was then that I realised how dangerous these so called religions were, and to this day I believe they should all be made illegal and outlawed. The train journey gave me time to reflect on the things that had happened to me on my travels. The only time I was really happy was when I was travelling, it made me forget. Hitchhiking was exciting and you had the freedom to go anywhere. The rest of my time away was an education and it taught me that it was not easy to survive without money. When I had lived rough, it was temporary and I also knew it but I knew that I would not have liked to live like that permanently.

Now I was heading home and I had to try and face my problems. My dreams were still there but I had to forget them for a while and try to build a life for myself. The 'Little Lady' I so yearned to meet was still a dream but I could not let it go, was it so much to ask? I had to try to hang on to the little faith in God I had left and everything would turn out right. Eventually!

The ferry crossing was good and I had enough money to have a drink, which I'd had so little of during the last few weeks. By the time I retired to my cabin I was well on the way to being inebriated!

The following morning I woke up to find we were approaching Harwich, so I just had time to eat some breakfast before disembarking.

It was raining when I took my first step on English soil for six weeks, and without looking back I strapped on my rucksack and went home!

ATIVAN AND BRICKS, ETC.

Nothing had changed at home and within a few days I had forgotten all about my travels. I felt miserable, but tried not to bother Mum with my problems. For once I had a reason to be depressed. I had no work, therefore no money, in fact I was in debt to Mum for the hundred pounds she sent me while I was away. I had dole money which paid for my keep and allowed me to go up to the Hen and Chickens for a couple of nights a week but I knew I had to find a solution, a way out of my difficulties before too long because my depression was getting worse.

Another problem was my stomach. I was getting almost incessant heartburn by now and that also affected me psychologically. The pressure was building up! I reached a stage when I could not take it any longer and one Saturday; about three weeks after I arrived home, it happened!

I was sitting indoors watching television when I felt what can only be described as a feeling of dread, with this came the terrifying feeling of sheer and utter panic. I ran into the kitchen and in tears told Mum that I could not take it anymore. This frightened Mum, and she stood there not knowing what to do and all I could say to her was, 'Please help me!'

Mum composed herself a little and tried to talk to me, but I was in such a state that her words were of little help to me. I begged her to call a doctor, which after failing to calm me down, she did. I went and sat in the dining room, in the quiet and tried to compose myself but had little success and all that seemed to help was pacing up and down the room. This I did for more than an hour, in fact, I did not stop until the doctor arrived. The doctor did not seem very sympathetic; in fact, he seemed a little annoyed at being called out for such a 'trivial' thing. I did not care; all I cared about was him doing something to alleviate the horrible feelings I had. I was desperate and let him know how desperate I was. He did give me something in the end and also told me to go and see the family doctor on Monday. Whatever he gave me seemed to calm me down but I was still in shock, so I felt unattached to the real world and also as the symptoms eased I began to feel really hungry, as well as very, very tired.

After eating a meal I went straight to bed and although greatly fatigued I found it difficult to sleep. The whole episode had frightened me and even with the medication I had taken I found it very hard to relax my mind. Eventually I dropped off, but I woke up several times during the night and by morning I began to feel panicky again.

I spent the Sunday quietly, took more of the tablets I had been given and sat in the lounge trying to concentrate on watching television. Mum and Tom seemed concerned for me and did their best to help. By bedtime the medication seemed to be doing its job and I began to feel a bit more human even though I was doped up.

On Monday morning Mum drove me to the surgery where I made an immediate appointment to see a lady doctor. While sitting in the waiting room I felt very on edge and vulnerable but tried to discipline myself to keep the feelings of panic under control. After I had been waiting for what seemed several hours I was finally told I was next to see the doctor. I went in and remained there for a good quarter of an hour trying to explain all the symptoms I had experienced over the last couple of days.

The doctor asked me about my life in general and said I needed more to occupy my mind and was reluctant to give me any more medication. I became very concerned when she said this, and anxious not to experience any more panic attacks. I virtually begged her for medication saying I could not get by without it. She succumbed to my pleading and prescribed the tranquilliser Ativan (Lorazepan).

Once back home I had a big discussion with my mother and she reiterated what the doctor had said. I knew they were both right and decided that once I had settled down I would try to sort my life out.

Within a week on medication I felt well enough to venture out to the Hen and Chickens and soon repeated this when my funds allowed. As I was feeling better all round I decided to try and contact Keith and Linda again. When I phoned them they were surprised and pleased to hear from me and said they did not realise I was back from my travels. They soon started taking me out again and this proved to be very therapeutic, although my underlying depression was still lingering.

It was about this time that a sinister complication in my mental health came to the surface. When I was around people, especially vulnerable ones, I had to fight off an apparent urge to lose control of myself and harm them. This upset me, because it was against my nature, but as it went on I tried harder and harder to fight it. This created another problem because I became afraid to stop fighting it in case I lost control. Thinking this way compounded the problem and increased my anxiety even more.

I realised that I had to tackle the problem and do it fast, to cut the anxiety level before it once again got out of control.

While in bed one night it suddenly dawned on me that I would not hurt anybody and the only way people harm other people was when they consciously plan it and premeditate it. So I told myself that instead of fighting my fear I should ignore it.

In the following days I tried out my theory and discovered that it worked. It did not stop the thoughts that lead to the fear, but it suppressed it rather than compounding it. Although I had found the solution the only real way to suppress the unwanted thoughts was through drink only then could I really relax and free my mind.

My trips to the doctor became regular and as time passed I found it increasingly difficult to obtain my prescription for more Ativan. In the end, roughly five months after my initial visit, the doctor arranged an appointment for me to see a psychiatrist at the nearby hospital and at the same time arranged another appointment to try and sort out my stomach problems. The psychiatrist's appointment came first but proved to be a complete waste of time. Firstly the person I saw was a Polish woman who was very hard to understand and secondly she only really told me what I knew already, and that was to socialise more and to get a job! The only real result I got out of the visit was that she recommended that I stay on Ativan for a further period (until I saw her again) and also prescribed some anti-depressants to help ease my blues. I did tell her about my illogical thoughts but she did not seem at all concerned. After a few weeks my depression eased and I began to feel slightly better but I was still troubled with unwanted thoughts and developed the theory that Ativan was to blame, so I made a conscious effort to cut down my intake of them and only to take one when really necessary. It did not seem to help, so I had to learn to live with the thoughts. I saw the psychiatrist once more and she took me off the anti-depressants, she was pleased with my progress especially as I had cut down the Ativan and did not wish to see me again!

The appointment for my stomach check-up came along and involved drinking a Barium Meal so they could see any problems on a scanner. It was not very pleasant drinking the stuff because it was so thick and heavy and you could feel it going through your system.

When I returned home the Barium Meal had already completed its journey so I had to make a quick visit to the toilet. Afterwards Mum had to spend some time unblocking the toilet pan as the contents were too heavy to flush away.

By now we were well into 1981 and I was starting to look forward to getting my driving licence back at the end of May. My work situation was still unpromising and I was beginning to wonder if I would ever work again. My mental health remained a problem, but I continued taking Ativan when I needed it so I was able to control my anxiety or so I thought at the time.

One night down the Hen and Chickens I was talking to a man I had not seen before and very soon the conversation turned to work. I told him I was unemployed and had previously worked in the building trade. He asked me if I could do plastering as he had some that needed doing at home. Being honest I told him that I had never before attempted such work but had watched it being done many times and would be willing to try it. He replied that he would be willing to let me do the job but would only pay me if he was happy with the result. I thought that was fair enough, so after agreeing that he would buy the materials we shook hands on the deal.

When I told Mum about the job she seemed very pleased and commented that it might lead to other things. With this in mind, I caught the bus to nearby Woking and purchased the necessary tools I needed to carry out the work. The following day, tools in hand, I set off for the work not really knowing what to expect.

There were only two small walls to be plastered but it took me the best part of the day to complete them. It was work I did not enjoy but I stuck at it and when I had finished I thought I had done a reasonable job. My new friend (the owner) surveyed the newly plastered walls and remarked that for my first time they were pretty good. He paid me for the work and then said he would like a patio laid at the back of the house and was I interested? Of course I said, 'Yes'! This time he wanted me to quote a price, something that I found very difficult, but again I only had to price for labour so it was not that difficult.

At home that evening I excitedly told Mum about the day and told her that after doing the patio I would be able to buy some transport, and once I had my licence back (now within a month) things were bound to pick up. It took a long time to sleep that night as I was excited about various thoughts that had come to me. They all involved work and money. When I received my licence back I would buy a small van and put an advertisement in the local paper advertising my services as a small builder and take on any small jobs that came my way whether or not I had tackled similar ones before!
In the morning I told Mum my plan and, although pleased, she warned me to be careful. The same morning I went to see the doctor to get more Ativan and hear about my results of the stomach scan. I was told that I had developed a duodenal ulcer, but not to worry because a new drug was on the market. The drug was called Tagamet and I was given a prescription for them.

After a few days, while laying the patio, I managed to get some more plastering work off another man I knew, so I was booked up with work until I had my licence back!

Although I was being paid cash at that time I realised the future need to become self-employed, so I sent away for all the necessary forms in preparation. Within a fortnight of 'licence day' I put an advertisement in the paper and started looking for a suitable vehicle. The day came and, with my new driving licence and second-hand Morris Minor van and a list of potential clients, I really felt I was, at last, going somewhere! The same week I signed off the 'Dole' and registered self-employed. Now I would have to succeed!

Although I had work and consequently more money I still felt low and lethargic. My fear of losing control still haunted me and it was a daily battle to keep it under control. Also, as a consequence of acquiring a vehicle, the fear of steering into oncoming traffic returned, especially on longer journeys. Despite these problems I continued to take Ativan and continued to believe that that was causing them. I also continued to believe that my depression was due to the lack of a relationship in my life.

My social life consisted mainly of visiting the Hen and Chickens which became part of daily routine. Every now and then, mostly at weekends, I drove over to Weybridge where Keith and Linda lived and perhaps would spend the night. It always tended to be a boozy couple of days, but normally enjoyable.

It was now summertime and when Sue came to stay we once again started to plan a holiday together. We decided on going to France, but this time we would drive over there in my van! There were various doubts expressed about the van's reliability but I was very confident that it would tackle any journey asked of it.

My confidence was justified because the two weeks we were away it never let us down once and considering the amount of miles we did, it did us proud.

While in France, we visited St Malo and stayed on a camp site for a couple of nights becoming friendly with a Dutchman who took a shine to Sue. After that we drove south and stayed at a camp site I had stayed at the previous year. Then, after a week in the sunshine and after striking up a friendship with a German couple, we headed home via the scenic route of eastern France.

All through the holiday my mind was on women. Unfortunately, as I have said before, when you are on holiday with your sister, everywhere you go people think you are a couple so it is extremely difficult to explain differently. Sue must have felt the same but did not say anything; nevertheless we had an enjoyable fortnight.

Once back home I became engrossed in work once more. The jobs I was getting were very varied and I was learning all the time. I built walls and patios, laid concrete paths, repaired roofs, laid drains, painted, and even turfed gardens. I taught myself everything about the building and allied trades and all my clients were very pleased with my work.

With my working life going nicely my social life needed improvement. I was still unhappy and yearned for a relationship. I began to spend more time with Keith and Linda again. Whereas before I would see them maybe once a fortnight, now I was out with them two or three times a week. The only problem was drinking and driving. I had learned my lesson since my ban and especially as I needed transport for my work.

Keith had been caught drink driving as I had, but

in his case it did not seem to make any difference, he still drank and he was still driving! Many times we were out drinking and many times Keith would drive home three sheets to the wind!

All through 1982 and into 1983 my life did not change, I was working hard and I was drinking hard. I was out every night either up the Hen and Chickens or with Keith and Linda.

I tried to stay out of Mum and Tom's hair as much as possible and started to look forward to getting a place of my own as I never felt really relaxed in Tom's company and we quite often crossed swords over really trivial matters. This put Mum in awkward positions but she was always as diplomatic as possible, trying not to take sides.

My relationship with Hazel did not improve either. She was as impossible as ever, therefore I carried on seeing very little of Dad. At this time whenever I did see him it was as if we were strangers and we almost had to get to know each other over again!

In February of 1983 I went on an unexpected holiday. A couple of brothers, who used the pub, had arranged a week's trip to the 'Algarve' in Portugal. One of their friends had dropped out at the last minute so they asked me if I would like to go. I agreed, although I was a bit dubious about the others going (eight in all) because I did not particularly feel at ease with groups of people, especially as I did not know them all.

My fears were justified because on the first night in Portugal we all went out for a meal and I found it extremely hard to join in the festivities and felt left out. Another factor about the evening was that it proved expensive and I spent a lot more than intended, leaving me with a tight budget for the rest of the week.

The following morning I was feeling a bit worse for wear (too much booze) so I went and sat on the beach. As I sat there I began to feel as though the beach was going to swallow me up and a very big sensation of claustrophobia engulfed me. I panicked and rushed off the beach imagining that I could not breathe.
Fortunately, I had the foresight to bring some Ativan on holiday with me so I rushed up to the hotel room and took some, after which I sat on the edge of the bed until I felt better.

The rest of the holiday I refrained from drinking and spent most of it by myself, mainly because I felt so fragile and wanted to remain as quiet as possible. The others, I am sure thought I was being extremely unsociable, but I knew I needed peace and quiet so I had little choice in the matter.

The last two days of my excursion to Portugal seemed at first to be a matter of survival. I wandered around the resort aimlessly, trying to forget my fragile state. My intake of Ativan was higher than it had ever been but I did not care, just as long as I made it home in one piece. I did not tell any of the others how I was feeling, for one thing I felt ashamed of myself and for another I knew I would get little sympathy.

Then, out of the blue, I met someone who transformed my remaining time into very precious moments. Up until that moment my sex life had been virtually non-existent and my eternal quest for love had made me forget about the physical side of a relationship, although, of course, I still had fantasies. The young lady I met was what I could only call a gift from God.
I was wandering around the local market when I decided to buy an apple. While at the stall I noticed a girl

purchasing some fruit and speaking English, she was quite short with medium length dark brown hair and had a figure that caught my eye straight away. Without thinking I just said 'hello' to her, she turned towards me and with a broad smile returned the greeting. Again with equal abandonment I asked her if she would like to go for a coffee. She said, 'Yes'.

It all happened so quickly that I could hardly believe it when we were sitting opposite each other drinking coffee. As usual I was honest with her, her being Julie, and I told her I was going through a bad time at the moment, but she seemed to take it in her stride. After coffee we walked along the beach and talked some more. She told me that she had been in Portugal for some time and I asked her if she liked the men, to which she replied she liked most men. She then said something that I could not believe at first, so I made her say it again and that was and I quote, 'The trouble with me is that I like sex so much'. After the initial shock, I told her that I quite liked it myself and should we go to her apartment and talk about it.

The next 24 hours were out of this world and although I still had to take Ativan, I still had the best time of my life. Julie was insatiable and very accommodating, there was nothing she would not do and I was a very willing partner for her.

After the initial lust, we had a shower together and went to the local casino but did not win anything. When we returned to her apartment we resumed where we had left off and made love several times before we both collapsed into bed and fell asleep.

The following morning there was no time for even breakfast, because I had to rejoin the others and go to the airport to return home. We said our goodbyes and Julie wished me well and hoped I would soon be better, and I told her to be careful. I wished that I could have stayed longer, but deep down knew it was better that way, so we parted with a kiss and that was all!

The memory of Julie slowly disappeared into the back of my mind, but even today I wish I could relive those 24 hours but this time not to be drugged up to the eyeballs!

After a few days of being home I settled down again and my consumption of Ativan dropped considerably although I still took it when necessary. It helped my overall mood and it helped to control the fears and anxieties I experienced. I still believed that when I met a girl and fell in love I would be able to do without any medication at all!

Work was going well even though I found every job a chore and did not enjoy any aspect of it at all. But I stuck to it and still took pride in it and I was getting more and more work through word of mouth. Soon after coming back from Portugal I was in a position to get rid of my old van, which had served me well, and purchase a brand new Datsun pick-up truck. I did not buy it outright but put down a deposit on it and agreed to pay a monthly sum over three years.

To coincide with my new transport I decided I was in a position to call myself a builder, so I had a sign on the truck to say so. I also changed my advertisement in the local paper to include building extensions. I had already thought of a business name for myself, it was 'Philip Westam' and my business sign was in Claret and Blue! Yes, I still supported West Ham United.
When I had time to sit back and view things, I felt proud when I realised how far I had come in just two years. I think Mum was proud as well, although my mental

health was still on her mind.

Apart from word of mouth, I used to get many enquiries about work over the phone. As my diary filled up I was in a position to pick and choose what job I undertook. I still used to price any job I was asked to, but not all of them realistically, in other words any job I did not fancy I would price higher so if I did get it, it would be well worth doing.

On one occasion I had a phone call from a man called Peter Neal who was a painter and decorator. He told me he had many jobs that required building work to be done and was I interested in doing them? After careful consideration I decided to meet Peter and discuss terms. He was a very likeable chap who was in his forties and had a very impressive client list. His clients were very wealthy people and included a few celebrities, Bruce Forsyth to name just one. He also told me that he was a carpenter by trade, which I thought would be useful to me.

From that point onwards we became friends and helped each other out as much as possible. Early on in our relationship I found working with Pete was a lot more enjoyable than working by myself and I found myself even waking up and not finding it an effort getting out of bed!

As I was working hard, time went quickly and before I had a chance to draw breath we were into 1984. By now, despite taking little Ativan, my fear of hurting people was still prevalent, in fact it was getting worse and I was finding it increasingly difficult to rationalise. I faced the dilemma of taking more Ativan (which I thought was the source of my problem) to alleviate my increasing anxiety or remain on a small dose and put up with the now very big problem of my negative fears. I decided to increase my dosage of the drug and see what happened.

After a couple of weeks I certainly felt better and looked at the world with renewed hope for my future. Further hope came from an unlikely source. While I was still seeing Keith and Linda I got to know Linda's mother quite well and occasionally she would give me a further reading of the future but none of them seemed to compare to the first one she had given me. One day I was in her company once again when we were talking about things in general. I told her that I was not feeling particularly well and had not done so for some time. She then went on to tell me about her connection with the spiritualist church and how there were healers within the church who often helped people with their ailments.

From that time on I became interested in spiritual matters and sometimes attended church meetings in Woking. The Sunday services were very different from orthodox churches and had a medium giving messages from the spirit world instead of a sermon. After a short while I began to think that maybe there was a connection between my problems and the spirit world, although I had no idea what!

One day, while at a service I was introduced to a healer and after a short chat she invited me to the healing sessions she practised on Wednesday evenings. I decided I had nothing to lose so I went along and it soon became a regular thing. The reason why it became a regular thing was because it was so peaceful in the church and while the healer 'did her stuff' I used to become very warm and relaxed, although in general my problems remained the same.

I carried on going to the healing sessions for a good few

weeks and even tried to drag Mum along, but to no avail. One Wednesday evening I went along to the church as usual and bumped into a medium at the entrance. It was unusual to see her on a Wednesday evening, so I asked her why she was there. She said that she was going to perform a very important exorcism, and then, with my prompting went into further detail.

Apparently there was a young Asian girl who was possessed by a troubled spirit, which had to be removed and she (the medium) was going to use her own body (with the help of other mediums) to do this.

On hearing this I became fascinated and scared at the same time. When I sat down for my healing session I could hear everything that was going on in the next room, so I listened intently. My healing session abandoned, I became transfixed by the events next door. I could hear the medium's voice as she spoke to the girl. She started by telling her not to be frightened and to try to relax, then she started talking to the spirit and tried to draw it out of the girl's body and into her own. She succeeded, and immediately it became so, the spirit started to speak through her and the voice I heard was very different from the medium's. It was very frightening to listen to and very hard to describe except to say that it made my hair stand on end.

At that point the two other mediums started trying to persuade the spirit to leave this world and move towards the bright light it should be able to see. It took a lot of persuasion but eventually the spirit left the medium's body and went on into the next world.

Afterwards when everything returned to normal I wanted to speak to the medium who had let herself be used by the spirit, but she had already left. There was, however, still one of the other mediums in the church so

I spoke to him and remarked about the voice I had heard. He said the voice was nothing and if that frightened me it was a good thing that I never saw her face!

It was not long after that evening that I realised that the healing (although pleasant at the time) was not doing much good, so my visits to the church became a rarity and as my problems increased dwindled out altogether. I never forgot what I had learned at the spiritualist church and even now base my beliefs on those teachings.

As I mentioned before, I was still occasionally seeing Keith and Linda but as the summer of 1984 came along they started growing apart. I had sensed something was wrong for quite a while and often had chats with Keith, but he was a person who never opened up at the best of times so I just waited for the inevitable to happen. They split up very abruptly and before I knew where I was I was having a drink with Keith one night when out of the blue he told me. That night he also told me he would stay in touch with me but I never saw him again. I often wonder what happen to him, because he seemed very confused and distant when I last saw him and I was a bit concerned about him. Both he and Linda were good friends to me and I felt a big sense of loss when they were finally gone and life without them took a bit of getting used to.

Up until then I had never had a long relationship, but then something happened out of the blue to change that. One day I ran into an old friend who I knew from my days at the hospital social club and we got talking. She told me that she now shared a flat in Guildford and was having a party the next Saturday night and I was welcome to go along.

Not being the best of party goers I had more or less

decided not to go, but as Saturday approached I became very bored with going up the Hen and Chickens every night and decided I needed a break. I was very apprehensive at first, even before I set off for Guildford, but once I was there I relaxed a little. There were not that many people at the flat, but it still seemed pretty crowded because it was not very big. As I circulated (by the drinks table) I got talking to my friend's flat mate, who was a girl about my age called Pam. As we talked I began to feel calm, much calmer than usual when I talked to girls. Before long we were dancing together and for the first time in my life I realised that I had been picked up!

As the evening wore on and Pam had gone to the loo, I wondered whether I should take the opportunity and leave. Although Pam was a nice girl to talk to I did not particularly fancy her (which was probably the reason I was so calm) and really did not know if I wanted to sleep with her. I decided to have another drink and stay because by now I had had too many to drive home anyway.

This was the start of our relationship and it lasted about six weeks. There is not much more to say about it because we were a very ordinary couple and did very little socialising apart from the odd drink out together. We made love regularly, mostly at the flat but there was one night when Pam stayed at mine and I crept into her bedroom for a 'quick one'. Sex was the only thing I got out of the relationship, that and feeling at ease with her, which was becoming harder for me to do with everyone.

As we came to the end of our relationship it became very evident that Pam was in love with me, which made it harder for me to break it off. I ended it abruptly!

It was over quicker than I thought mainly because

I expected Pam to ring me for an explanation, but she never did. She was a lot braver than I would have been in the same situation and my heart went out to her hoping she did not suffer too much. To this day I remember her as the only girl who really loved me.
It was not long after Pam that the shoe was on the other foot. I was still using the Hen and Chickens regularly (almost every night) and getting my therapy out of a glass when I began to notice a young lady more and more. She was heavily pregnant at the time so I more or less convinced myself that I would be wasting my time with her. I adopted that attitude, however the lady in question started to notice me and would often smile at me and look in my direction. Of course, I began to reciprocate the attention and was often caught in the act by her husband!

    It soon started to get embarrassing and I decided to drink in the other bar to avoid an imminent confrontation. It did not stop there though because the lady used to go to the loo regularly which meant walking past me. Every time she passed me she would look at me and smile. By this time I was besotted!

    Every minute of the day I spent thinking about this lady and I thought at last I had found my true love. It got to the stage that I did everything to avoid looking at her because I was becoming obsessed with her and I knew it could possible get out of control. One day I decided that I had to do something to put me out of my misery, so I poured out my heart in a letter which I would give her at the next possible moment.

    My moment came very shortly after she had had her baby. She obviously had to stay at home to look after it, so one evening I made sure her husband was in the pub and I delivered the letter to her at home (I had previously found out her address). I had never been so nervous in my life but I knew it had to be done. When she answered the door I was stumped for words so I just thrust the letter to her and ran off back down the drive!

I never had a reply or a phone call or anything and to rub in what a fool I was, her husband started to take the Mickey out of me with a number of friends one night up the pub. She had obviously shown him the letter. I did not see much of her after that, but a year later I heard she had split up with her husband. On reflection I realised that again I had become too heavy too quickly and hated myself for it.

Towards the latter part of 1984 I was very busy and earning lots of money, so I was able to save a fair bit. I still, however, did not enjoy my work and every morning was a battle to motivate myself and get ready for the day's work. When things went wrong, and as the time past increasingly so, I became very stressed up and tended to blame myself for every mishap. I really did not like myself and even when the job had finished and I could stand back and look at what I had achieved, I never gained a sense of pride or congratulated myself on a job well done. One big factor in my favour when working was my undying determination to finish the job and to do it to the highest standards whatever the cost. One job I started at this time was the biggest project I had ever tackled. It was a double-sized carport complete with a sloping roof and built in a style to match the existing house. It took six weeks to build and with the help of Peter Neil, who made a good job of the roof, it impressed the client immensely and enhanced my reputation no end. After that I thought I had more than earned the right to call myself a builder!

With plenty to do on the work front and bored with

my life I developed an interest in Car Boot Sales. To start with I used to visit various events at the weekend, but as time passed I began to purchase various items at what I thought bargain prices and keep them until I had enough to set up my own stall and resell them.

As a beginner I did not always make a profit, but I was learning all the time and eventually I started to specialise in certain things. My biggest speciality was paperbacks books. Many people sold a few paperbacks, but mainly they asked very low prices so I recognised the opportunity of money to be made. I designed and made special book cases and filled them with books at realistic prices and made a fair bit of money at it. I used to replenish my stocks by arriving early and going round other stall holders and buying up all the bargains. I liked making money that way and even started to enjoy myself sometimes, which was a rarity in those days.

As the year came to an end I was extremely busy and had little time to think about myself. I was still taking Ativan and still fighting the negative fears I had developed, but they had almost become part of my life, although I still fought against them all the time. I was determined that my life would not be taken over by any thoughts that should not be there, and while I could rationalise I could keep a tight rein on them!

Christmas was looming again, but Christmas 1984 was to turn out especially significant.

Tom had been moved again. He was going to work back in Norwich which meant moving house and trying to build a new life back near where Sue and I spent our final school years. Sue, of course, was still living and working in Norfolk and was delighted with the news whereas I had work commitments in Surrey and felt settled there. There was no question really that I would stay in Surrey, but where would I live!

My final Christmas with all the family in Surrey was very enjoyable and exciting because I had decided that I had enough money to put down a deposit on a house of my own. I was at last going to leave the family home and at the age of 27 became completely independent for the first time in my life.

After a lot of searching I found a house that I felt was suitable. It was situated on a very big estate between Woking and Knaphill called Goldsworth Park and was only a couple of miles from Bisley, so I could still use the Hen and Chickens and stay in touch with the people I knew. The house also had the potential to be extended because some of the others in the cul-de-sac had already added on an extra bedroom and garage.

For once in my life everything went like clockwork and I was able to move into my new abode a couple of weeks before Mum and Tom moved to Norfolk. A lot of people were good to me. I was given a bed and a three-piece suite and managed to get carpets from a job I was doing with Peter Neil. A lot of the other things like crockery and kitchen utensils I managed to purchase at Car Boot Sales. Mum was very good to me by supplying curtains and linen, while I bought a fridge and cooker from a local paper.

There was so much happening in my life in the New Year of 1985. I started a new job, my first extension. I had also fallen in love again, with the wife of my new client. Her name was Julie and I took to her the first time I saw her. She knew how I felt - it was written all over my face, but at first she pretended not to let me know it. As the job progressed and I saw more of her I started to sense that she liked me too and there were a few times when we were talking that I could barely contain myself from grabbing hold of her and kissing her, but I never did. I still do not know the real reason why I did not try it on, maybe it was because I liked her husband or maybe it was because they had a wonderful little baby or maybe I was just plain scared. Whatever the reason I continued to love her and for once I looked forward to going to work each morning.

I was seeing someone else at the time, a young lady called Sarah who I met down at the Hen and Chickens. She was not particularly my type but it was nice to think that I had a companion for once. I did not see her more than about twice a week and I was not really sure whether I could call her my girl friend or not. She used to play me around a lot and I did most of the running (as usual), so most of the time I was feeling unhappy and frustrated. I knew there was no future in our relationship but at that moment in time I was feeling particularly vulnerable and could not seem to break it off.

One night I was sitting in my new home feeling lonely when somebody rang the door-bell. I opened the door and found that it was Sarah. She had one thing on her mind and that was sex! I was very surprised at first because we had not made love since we met (about three weeks), although it was not for through lack of trying on my part.

We went up to the bedroom and both naked, jumped into bed, that's when disaster struck! I could not relax my mind and concentrate on the job in hand; whatever I did I could not make it. It was so frustrating for both of us and ended with Sarah jumping out of bed, dressing and storming out of the house. I implored her to stay but she would not listen, I never saw her again.

In the morning I felt devastated and sat in the chair downstairs and started to cry. In my desperation I said a prayer and pleaded with God to let her ring me. It was a prayer so deep and full of emotion that I still remember it to this day.

What happened next was something very strange, because as I stopped praying and tried to compose myself, the phone rang. I picked up the receiver and after saying, 'Hello' listened for a reply. I must have listened for a good 10 seconds, but met with only silence until finally there was a click at the other end.

Most people would have put my phone call down to coincidence and thought it was done as a hoax, but I took more notice of it and was proved right, as you will learn as you read on. I received quite a few similar calls from then on, some of them at insignificant times, but a few I received were very significant as you will see!

My love for Julie did not diminish, in fact if anything increased, and right up until the end of my work at hers I used to think about her a lot. Thoughts of her started to become an obsession and started to increase my mental health problems, so I tried mostly unsuccessfully, to think of other things. The problem was that she continued being warm towards me especially when things were not going so well with the job. When I was upset she used to bring me a cup of tea and sit talking to me while I drank it.

One night I was feeling particularly lonely and I had gone to bed early, I started to fantasising about Julie, although that was not unusual in itself, this night my thoughts were very deep and I got so involved that I almost thought she was with me in bed and I began to feel very warm and relaxed. I could not sustain the intensity of my thoughts at that level indefinitely however and eventually came down to earth, but it was a magical feeling while it lasted. As I lay there immediately afterwards, the phone rang and once again there was nobody on the other end, but I listened to the silence and it went on for ages before the familiar click and the purring sound. Then I went to sleep.

Most nights I was very tired, not just physically but emotionally as well and any night that I turned in without having a drink I used to have to take Ativan to relax my mind. I started to have fears that I was an alcoholic and could sleep only after having a drink. My overall anxiety level became very high in this period; it became so high that I could not function at work properly. Julie seemed to notice my problems increasing, and was worried about me suggesting that it would be wise to see my doctor.

Taking Julie's advice, I made an appointment with my local doctor. My stomach was playing up again, so I told him about it and he recommended that a specialist at the hospital should see me and have what was called an endoscopy. As for my anxiety, he said that I was taking on too much and that I should lighten the load a little. Also he suggested I take a regular high dose of Ativan for a while until I got sorted out.

After contemplation, I decided that I would take on a labourer which would make my life a lot easier, and besides I could afford one. So that is what I did. I took on a young West Indian lad called Philip who proved to be a very good worker, despite coming to work every day stoned! Apart from smoking dope, he used to work all day with reggae blasting his ears off on his personal stereo!

Philip was like a ray of sunshine to me, he

certainly brightened up my life with his 'couldn't care less attitude' and very sharp sense of humour. I kept him on until Julie's extension was finished, and when I laid him off I promised that if I needed another labourer I would certainly get in touch. It was a wrench to say goodbye to Julie, but I told her to ring me anytime for a chat or if she needed any more work done. I did not hear from her nor had I really expected to, but carried on loving her for a long time.

After finishing the extension I took a couple of weeks off. It certainly did me some good although I still had to take Ativan, but I fought against it as usual. By now I felt isolated and out of touch with the real world and I knew something was badly wrong with me and I racked my brains to try to fathom out what it was. As I improved slightly from my rest I once again put my problems down to the side effects of the Ativan and the lack of a relationship. I seemed incapable of thinking logically about my symptoms and used to sit for hours trying to sort my thoughts out before returning to where I had started. When I was with people I spent all my time fighting the fear of losing control and hurting them while when I was driving I was fighting the fear of losing control of the car, this gave me little time to think of many other things. One thing I never stopped believing was that I was strong enough to keep my fears at bay. My appointment for the hospital came up and although my stomach was a little better, after the doctor put me back on Tagamet (which I had taken previously), I still decided to keep the appointment. I was in hospital all day while they put me out and pushed a mini camera down into my stomach. The worst bit was coming round in the middle of the proceedings and starting to choke and trying to pull the camera out before they increased the anaesthetic and I slipped under again.

They told me the results before I went home and said that there had been ulcers but the medication had cleared them up, so the best thing to do was to stay on Tagamet to keep the symptoms at bay. I knew myself that smoking was probably to blame, but also knew that at that moment in time I could not possibly give up.

After finishing Julie's extension I decided to knuckle down and start work on my own house. I had already submitted plans to the council and they had, as expected, given the go ahead. My next door neighbour had, after discussing it with me, decided to extend his house at the same time. We agreed that if I provided all the labour he would buy all the materials for both jobs. So, with everything sorted out, I started work.

As I wanted to concentrate on the work at home I signed on the unemployment list and started receiving Income Support and got help with my mortgage as well. I had a bit of money saved up and decided that it could be used for my less frequent trips to the Hen and Chickens, and a holiday within a few weeks. So with no money problems I got stuck into the very large project I had landed myself with!

By September I had made significant progress and the extensions were coming on well. I was so pleased that I had decided to take my holiday then. My anxiety level seemed stable at that time, mainly because I had been careful not to put myself under undue pressure, but nevertheless I felt I needed a holiday. I booked a late bargain to Spain's Costa Del Sol and within two weeks I was on the plane, full of optimism and again wondering if this would be the trip where at last I found happiness. I had purposely chosen a Scandinavian Hotel as I still had it in my mind that my destiny lay with Scandinavian people.

When I arrived at the hotel I found that I had been booked to share a room with an elderly man who was half blind. I was not too happy with the situation but realised that I would have to put up with it. My room mate was a nice old boy and like all elderly people soon slipped into a routine, so I quickly got to know when he was about and when he was not!

The first week (I was there for two) in the daytime I spent the time basking in the sun by the pool and it was not long before I started to get to know people. Funnily enough the people I became friendly with first were English. They also enjoyed staying within the hotel grounds by the pool and once the early evening brought cooler weather we stayed out in the sunshine and enjoyed a drink together.

It was very relaxing at that time of the day, when most people had gone to prepare for dinner while we all sat there getting slowly drunk! By the time we had to go and prepare for the evening we were just nicely merry and ready for the dinner after a shower of course.

My English friends went home after three days so my holiday was altered. I soon came to miss them and especially our evenings together, but they were replaced by a Danish family who I got to know. This was because I fancied their daughter whose name was Gitte, she had been sitting by the pool one afternoon by herself and I unusually had the courage to speak to her. As I became friendly with her, I met her parents, and we soon became friends and I spent the rest of the first week mostly in their company.

I had a rival for Gitte's affection, a German guy. He was quite a friendly chap but I sussed him out straight away. The matter was resolved very quickly when Gitte's father asked me to go with them for dinner one evening in Torremolinos. From then on I spent a very pleasant few days in Gitte's company and was saddened when it was time for her to leave, although we did not even kiss, yet alone anything else. Despite not being intimate I developed a genuine affection for Gitte and remember her and her parents for contributing to what would be the last holiday and time that I ever really enjoyed.

With Gitte gone my holiday did not fall flat however, because I had previously arranged a meeting with Dad who just happened to be holidaying in the same region as me. I had also hired a car so it was easy for me to get around. I met up with Dad and Hazel (unfortunately) a little further along the coast where we went for a drink round one of his friends.

With my confidence higher than usual, and feeling tanned and fit, I found conversation easy and soon got talking to another Danish girl who was at Dad's friends place. I got on so well with her that it seemed inevitable that we would see each other again. Before leaving I made a date to see her the following day and promised to take her for a drive in the Spanish countryside.

When I arrived back at the hotel I spent the afternoon by the pool, staying there until early evening when I returned to my room to have a shower and get ready for dinner. I had just finished my shower when there was a knock on the door. As soon as I opened the door my latest 'Danish Pastry' walked in without saying anything and went and sat on my bed. Aware that my room mate was due anytime I felt it too risky to start what she obviously wanted me to do, so I had to tell her that I shared the room. She seemed to understand, so we talked for a while until my room mate arrived at which time she left saying that she would see me tomorrow. I felt very annoyed that I had lost the chance for a bit of fun and hoped upon hope that the next day would offer more opportunity.

The next day was quite enjoyable, but very hot sitting in the car for a lot of the time. We had lunch by a lake and my thoughts turned to sex but there were other people about so it proved impossible at that time, so I suggested that we went further round the lake but she said it was too hot and wanted to return to base. When we got nearer home I asked her back to my room saying that my room mate would not be there, but for some reason she declined. I arranged to meet her in the evening but she never turned up, so that was the end of that!

On an outing the following day (which I had booked in advance), I met an English girl who I rather fancied and we met for a drink that night. After downing 'quite a few' we went back to my hotel. As my room mate was in bed we made love in the dining room amongst all the made up tables, at one point we were making so much noise that we were lucky we were not caught!

I continued seeing the English girl for the rest of the holiday and introduced her to Dad, but all the time I knew she had a boy friend back home and there was no future for us anyway because we lived too far apart, but it was fun while it lasted.

The last few days of the holiday were spent relaxing by the pool in the early autumn sunshine and my thoughts turned to the previous few days. It seemed a lifetime since I had met Gitte and her parents. She was the girl I had grown attached to more than any other and ironically I had not even kissed her. Every one of the days on that holiday had been worth remembering and even today I think of those first few evenings lying by the pool in the company of new friends, drinking and watching the sun go down. I also remember the calmness and self-assurance I felt in myself and the eagerness with which I tried to reach out and grab every piece of happiness I could. Thank you God for giving me those two weeks.

The extensions to the two houses continued to take shape, slowly and much to my surprise my neighbour kept coming forward with the money for the materials. I was still doing work for Peter Neil now and again, but I was finding it harder and harder to motivate myself to do any type of work. As time went by my enthusiasm about the extensions dwindled into insignificance and a depression that I had never experienced before engulfed me and severely handicapped me in everything I tried to do.

It was not long before I fell out with Peter over my inability to complete a minor task and leaving the job incomplete. I just felt that I was mentally incapable of finishing the job to my own high standards. By now I was starting to feel that there was something, either the medication I was taking or maybe something more sinister wrong with me. I knew if I carried on working I would have a complete nervous breakdown.

Just a couple of months after returning from Spain I decided to take another fortnight's rest and in that time go to the doctor's again. The doctor again told me I was working too hard and recommended that I try a different medication from Ativan, namely Valium and a different sedative for night time. He also told me to make sure that I took them regularly.

For the whole fortnight I took Valium at the stated

dose but disregarded the other sedative. Within a few days I started to feel more rested for whatever reason, but still felt ill and short tempered. I kept myself to myself as much as possible and only ventured out to visit the pub most evenings. I was still using the Hen and Chickens at this time. I used to cycle there and back so I could not get stopped for drink driving again. However, one evening I was having a drink when the barmaid said something that upset me and I just flew off the handle, eventually ending up arguing with the landlord and storming out. That was the last time I visited the Hen and Chickens and with it went all the friends and acquaintances I had made and met throughout the years. By the time I started working again I was well aware that my life was falling apart and I seemed powerless to stop it. Everything I did to counter my 'misfortune' seemed to fail miserably and this made me suspicious. I kept recalling the young girl in the Spiritualist Church who was possessed by an unhappy spirit and started to wonder if I had a similar problem or even being under the influence of a curse.

Finally, one evening I took a long hard look at myself and my life and decided to 'pull myself together' and be very positive in the future. This seemed to work quite well for a few weeks, as long as I made sure that I remained positive in outlook and fought against negative thoughts. I even had no time for the negative fears that had plagued me for so long, although they were still prominent in the back of my mind.

During this period of positiveness I finished the brickwork on both extensions and had started doing the roofs, which as I was on a roll did not take long at all. I also started using a different pub that was much closer to home than the Hen and Chickens, so all in all things were looking up. To cap everything someone I knew quite well asked me to do another extension, and after a little consideration I accepted it.

I started working on the new extension in the spring of 1986 and at first was full of enthusiasm but the weather was against me and it rained heavily day in and day out. Frustration set in and I started back on the slippery slope to oblivion. The way I felt must have rubbed off on my client because he started to find fault with the work I had done and eventually we had a big argument and he told me to collect my tools and leave. Consequently I had to suffer a couple of weeks of threats of being taken to court for breach of contract before he came to his senses and dropped them.

What happened was typical and was now becoming the norm, so it did not upset me as much as it would have done a few months back and I did not dwell on it but just carried on with the project at home.
Once again I let negativity creep its way back into my mind. So, once again, I tried to replace all the negatives with positives but this time I found it harder. It became a battle, probably because my life in general was full of negatives, but I struggled on. The main problem was that it took a lot of concentration and without it a lot of negative thoughts crept back into my mind almost immediately. I needed something positive to happen in my life to change the way I naturally thought. With this in mind I promised myself another holiday as soon as I had finished all the work at home. This seemed to work for a little while but the trouble was that everything was, as I said, negative and it was extremely hard to break out!

Things became desperate again; I started to get very anxious and in my desperation went back to the doctor who seemed powerless to help me except to put me back on Ativan. There was what seemed like no other choice for me but to take the medication and see what happened and if it did not work I would be in real trouble. I started off by taking double the normal dose for four days then as I felt easier reduced down to the normal dose which I took religiously for two weeks.

During that period, especially when I felt a little better I spent a lot of time thinking about my predicament and came to the conclusion that the medication did help me to think more positively and ease my depression. Coming to this conclusion gave me renewed hope because I knew that Ativan worked for me, so I could use it as a crutch when necessary or until my situation changed.

By early summer, in spite of my dubious mental state, I managed to complete the bulk of the work at home which only left the decorating and tidying up to do. I tried to stand back and admire what I had achieved but was met with a feeling of indifference and emotional confusion. Nevertheless, the fact that I had finished the bulk of the work eased a little of the pressure that was on me.

Again, at short notice, I booked a holiday. I decided to go back to the same hotel as the year before and hoped that I would enjoy it as much. I would, however, go with a large stock of Ativan and a wish to find the love of my life. The love that I so craved for and needed to bring back a bit of sanity into my life. Maybe at last I could put the past behind me and find a new beginning! I would make this holiday the best ever and prove to myself that I can be normal and happy, just like other people.

Stepping off the plane onto the warm tarmac of

Malaga airport felt extremely good, it felt like I was returning home instead of just visiting. When I reached the hotel nothing had changed, everything seemed familiar. I was given a room several floors up and was thrilled to find it was a double room and I had it to myself! Before unpacking I went onto the balcony for a look at the view, and as I looked I felt a strong sensation of fear and dizziness along with a very acute sense of dread that I would somehow lose control of myself and fall over the safety rail to my death. I somehow backed away from the edge and into the room again, but I still had that immense dread of being close to death and knew that I could not stay in that room. So, I picked up my belongings and fled downstairs to reception.

As luck would have it there was a spare room on the ground floor, but I was warned that it was small, dark and dreary. It turned out to be all those three things but at least I felt safe and that was a big plus for me.
The rest of the day I spent by the pool, just like old times, but as the sun started to go down I found I was the only one left, so feeling slightly vulnerable I went back to my room for a shower. After dinner I visited a few of the local bars, failing to strike up a conversation with anybody else for any length of time. As the evening wore on I started to feel very isolated and lonely and, as my medication was in my room, I decided to call it a night. After taking a couple of Ativan, I lay on my bed and expected to feel its comforting effects but instead all I felt was the unbearable feelings of isolation followed by sheer panic. This went on for what seemed hours, so I took a further two tablets and paced up and down the small room until my symptoms eased.

For the rest of the holiday I felt far from well and very, very fragile even with the help of Ativan. All I could think of was successfully completing my days in Spain and making it home.

I spent most days around the pool, but sometimes roamed the streets and beach hoping to meet a 'Little Lady' who I still thought would be my salvation. The lady I met was not particularly small, but proved to be a lifeline to me.

Three days into the holiday I was lying by the hotel pool when two girls sat down beside me. They were both English and both from Norwich, so it was not long before I was speaking to them. One of them, whose name was Kerry, was particularly sympathetic towards me and as we grew closer she told me that she had mental problems of her own as she was a manic-depressive.

Kerry and I became lovers and along with her friend spent evenings together until they returned home at the end of my first week on holiday. In my second week I struck up a friendship with a further two English women. They were very understanding and nursed me through the remaining days and nights until it was time for a relieved me to return home.

Waiting at the airport was an anxious affair. I had it in my mind that if I did not catch the fight I would die, and to make matters worse the plane's departure was delayed! I must have taken six tablets that day and they did not seem to have any effect. All I felt that whole day was acute anxiety with nothing easing it until I reached British soil.

When I settled back home I rang up Kerry in Norwich. By this time, after a little thought, I decided that I wanted her to come and live with me in Surrey. After speaking to her however, it was plain that she wanted to stay in Norfolk. Once again I was disappointed and frustrated, and alone.

By and large, being home settled me down and I was able to do a little decorating without my stress level hitting the roof. On my holiday I had more or less decided to give building a rest for a while and, with the work at home more or less finished, I started to look for alternatives. It was not easy and after a few weeks looking, all I could come up with was doing a milk round!

Feeling just about over Kerry I felt able to take on a new challenge, so with nothing to stop me I became a milkman! As usual I found communication with other people a problem and soon got into a few scrapes with my workmates.

Every morning, as you load up the milk onto the float, you are supposed to check to see if your order is all there. However, some mornings if I was late arriving I did not have time so consequently I did not know if my order was short. Having had an argument with a couple of blokes over my bread order one day, it led to them 'ripping me off' and not supplying all the milk. I was totally unaware of their actions until my round was audited and it was found to be £20 in arrears. By this time I was on the verge of leaving because I found the early mornings too demanding (I had to get up at five o'clock), so I decided to pay the money I owed and put it down to experience.

A couple of days before I left, the manager got attacked by an angry worker and, as I was next door, I heard the shouting and without any thought just dived into the room and pulled the man off the manager. He was so grateful that he returned my £20. When I remember the incident all I can recall is the way I was shaking and dashed to the toilet, eventually calming down about a half hour after the incident.

The other thing I remember about my life as a milkman was while out on my round I saw a limousine obviously going to a wedding. I looked at the bride in the back and recognised her as my old flame, Kate. I think she saw me because she looked in my direction, but even if she did she did not show it.

I had always thought I was over Kate but when I saw her that day in her wedding dress I felt deeply affected by it. At 29 years of age I felt so alone and wondered if I would ever meet anyone and get married. It was still the thing that I wanted most out of life and it still seemed such a remote possibility.

A short time before packing in the milk round I was offered another extension to do. It was nice and local and again it was for someone I knew. I gave it a lot of thought, especially as I wanted to finish my own house and then sell it. After discussing matters with the client, we came to an arrangement that I would work for him four days a week, which would give me time to work at home.

With everything settled I started work the week after I left the milk round. Right from the start I was under pressure and from a very early stage I knew I should not have started. Nevertheless I stuck at it, trying to ignore all the pressure and trying to overcome the one over riding fear I felt. My client had three wonderful children who were always interested in what I was doing. For a normal person this would not have been a problem but for me it meant a constant fight! With the children always in close proximity my fear of losing control was very prominent; it became such a problem that sometimes I would break out in a sweat through the high level of fear. Everyday I was faced with the very high level of stress and I felt like telling the children to clear off and leave me alone. But there was nothing I could do except soldier on and rely on my strength of character to see me through.

While I was at work, I noticed a very attractive young lady who used to call every week staying about an hour. I asked my client, who was a hairdresser, about her and he told me she was also a hairdresser and her name was Karen. After further enquiries I found out that she was divorced and advertised for work in the local paper. The following weekend I found her phone number in the paper and plucked up the courage to ring her to get my hair cut. She came round one evening in the week and only then did I really notice how attractive she was.

Apart from being pretty she had a wonderful figure and the best backside I had seen in years. I was smitten straight away! I told Karen that I had asked her round under false pretences and I just really wanted to take her out. She seemed delighted with the idea, so very soon we were dating.

The relationship started off very well and although she was a very sexy lady I never did anymore than kiss her for the first couple of weeks. It was then that she went cold on me and said she wanted time to think things over. I knew deep down that she had sensed something was not quite right with me and no matter how much I tried to relax I knew I had lost her.

This time I was deeply wounded and it took weeks to get over Karen. I felt sure, early on in the relationship that at last I had found someone, but once again I had lost out. One of the worst things that affected me was the fact that we never had sex together. She was the sexiest girl I had ever been with and looking back I remembered the many opportunities I had of seducing her but held back because I did not want to lose her. To this day I still have fantasies about Karen and try to imagine what might have been.

Unfortunately I saw Karen quite often after we had split up because she continued going round where I worked. This made it extremely difficult for me to get over her and doubly frustrating because I learned from my client that she was still looking for a partner, just like I was. One thing that I noticed at that time was the number of strange phone calls increased again and this added to my frustration, because every time the phone rang I was wishing that it was Karen and every time there was just silence.

To combat my feelings of loneliness and isolation I went to the local RSPCA kennels and got myself a dog. He was a white mongrel with black markings, round his eyes and I called him Charlie. However, right from the start he was more trouble than he was worth. The first day I had him he jumped over the fence at the back and disappeared for a few hours. He ran off at every available opportunity and I became more and more angry with him. More often than not I would get a phone call to say someone had got my dog (he had a tag on his collar with my phone number) and every time I used to have to fetch him, sometimes from the police station. One particular day Charlie ran off while I was at work and I arrived home feeling very tired when I had another phone call to say where he was. I jumped into my pickup and went to fetch him and I was very angry. When I got him I was so angry that I beat him hard a number of times before taking him home. That evening I had a visitor from an RSPCA officer after somebody had reported me for cruelty. This made me even angrier and once the officer had gone I lost my temper and started to yell my head off and throw things around, scaring Charlie to death. The officer had advised me to tie Charlie up, but I refused to admit defeat and decided instead to have him castrated. This I did and for a while he was much better, but it was not long before he was up to his old tricks again.

One evening I had a visitor and as I opened the door, Charlie escaped. He ran off up the road and disappeared leaving me, once again, frustrated and angry. He still had not returned when I went to bed, but at three o'clock in the morning I was woken by the telephone. When I picked up the receiver no one was there, but as I listened I could hear Charlie howling outside so I got up and let him in. Not all my strange phone calls were without meaning, occasionally they were relevant and were a warning and one particular one in the future that was to be of great help. I will tell you about that when the time comes.

My mental health was fluctuating from day to day and Charlie did not help. In the end I had to admit defeat and tie him up when he was out, otherwise if he continued running off I was afraid of what I might do to him. This was because my anger sometimes seemed uncontrollable and it scared me. Charlie was a very soft natured dog who loved affection and when he was out for a walk with me I would let him off the lead and he would never run off, always coming when called.

The extension I was doing at this time was the biggest I had ever tackled (except my own) and involved a lot of work. I promised myself that it would be my last, it was just too stressful. After making this decision I decided to celebrate by getting rid of my pickup truck and buying a car. Without thinking about the running costs I purchased a Rover SDI. It had all 'mod cons', including heated wing mirrors and automatic windows and sunroof. I was very proud of it and drove all over the place, getting used to its quick acceleration and power steering. It looked fine parked in front of my house and the neighbours all admired it. I went to Norfolk in it at the first possible moment and showed it to off to Mum, Tom and Sue and on the way back stopping in Essex to show Dad and Granddad. Granddad was very impressed! One thing I stipulated when I started on the final extension was that I would not work weekends. This enabled me to carry on doing the Car Boot Sales. During the many months in which I did them I met a lot of people, both male and female. One particular couple I had met had a unit in a mini market in Epsom where they sold tools during the week and on Saturdays. They approached me one Sunday and said that they were going away the following weekend and rather than shut the unit, would it be possible for me to look after it on the Saturday? I said that I would be pleased to.

So, on the Saturday In question, I sat and sold a few tools. It was not very busy and I became rather bored with it. While I was there I got talking to the girl on the refreshment bar. She was no oil painting but seemed to take to me, so feeling rather lonely I invited her back to my place for something to eat! One thing led to another and we ended up in bed. Once we had finished with the 'sexual activities' we got up and had something to eat.

After a meal we relaxed in front of the TV and to my surprise my latest friend started rolling a cannabis cigarette. Inevitably, she offered me one and as it was not the first time I took it. Everything seemed all right at first, but as I continued smoking I started to get very paranoid and only what can be described as a feeling that my mind was somehow detached from reality. As the minutes ticked by I felt more and more strange and I felt a very strong urge to scream my head off. Then I started to feel uncontrollable anger at my friend and had to use all my strength to stop myself attacking her for what she had given me. The only thing I could think of rationally was to grab my coat and go for a long walk until the drug had worn off. It was raining hard outside, but it did not deter me. While I walked I began to notice that every thought that came into my head seemed to take me over and became what seemed like reality. The more I thought about something the more the thought engulfed me. I tried to concentrate and think about good things but it was extremely hard to get rid of the previous thought from my head. I was very frightened by the whole episode and knew that I could not return home until I had walked it off. I must have walked for miles, although I never strayed far from home and it must have been two hours before I felt well enough to return to the warmth of the house.

Until then I had never felt that bad mentally and I vowed never again to touch anymore cannabis for the rest of my life. I thought of Karen and longed for her to come back into my life but, of course, she did not. Once again I wondered if I would ever find happiness instead the catalogue of disasters that I was experiencing. One thing I did notice was that the silent phone calls increased for a few weeks at this time.

Although I was working on the extension, I allowed myself enough time to get my house up to scratch. I longed to get the decorating finished as it was putting extra pressure on me and that was something that I could well do without. When I had completed painting the new bedroom I considered it as reaching a milestone because I could then use it. Once I had moved the furniture in I did a very silly thing. As the room still smelt of paint I lit a candle and placed it in a saucer and left it on the bedside table, hoping that it would remove the smell. I then forgot all about it and went for a drink up the pub.

On my return I was alarmed to find the house full of smoke and realising why, I dashed upstairs and cautiously opened the bedroom door. Apart from dense smoke there was nothing else to see, so I quickly opened the window and went downstairs and waited for the smoke to clear. Later after inspecting the room I considered how lucky I had been. The bedroom table was virtually non-existent, the telephone had disintegrated along with the radio/alarm and there was a big hole in the carpet. The bed which was only a foot away was undamaged. All I can imagine happened was that the dense smoke suffocated the fire before it could spread.

I was devastated at what had happened and cried with frustration, but I was more determined than ever to redecorate and finish the house. The insurance paid for the clean up and redecoration and I wasted no time in starting the work and within a month of the fire the house was finished.

Finishing my house did make a difference to the way I felt mentally although the effects of my success would not, I felt, be properly noticed until I had finished the other extension I was working on. Nevertheless, I decided that a move was in order so I put my house up for sale.

I did not intend moving far and indeed found a property that had the potential to develop in Bagshot, which was only seven miles away. All I had to do was to find a buyer for my house and I was in business. I did not have to wait long. Within two weeks of putting it on the market I sold it at a handsome profit! The money I had made was enough to buy the house in Bagshot and there was enough over to buy materials for an extension. The move went smoothly and I hoped against hope that the change would herald a new beginning for me. My new home was a cottage style semi and had a very long narrow kitchen which I planned to extend widthways; I also planned to put in a downstairs loo. The house, I noticed when I moved in, had a good atmosphere and for a few days I felt a sense of peace, a feeling that I had not felt for a long, long time. Charlie took a longer time to settle and was not happy. He got into the habit of tipping the rubbish out in the kitchen when I left him alone. Many nights, when returning from the pub, I would find him sitting amongst the rubbish strewn all over the floor. I tried everything to stop him doing it and was successful some of the time, but eventually I conceded defeat and for his safety more than anything else I returned him to the RSPCA.

It was not just Charlie I was short tempered with. Sue came to stay with me for a weekend and I remember giving her a really hard time, in fact I reduced her to tears. It was selfish but I did not seem capable of stopping myself which worried me immensely, as well as the rest of the family. To this day I regret hurting my sister because she was going through a difficult period in her life at that time and I made her feel even worse. I slipped from crisis to crisis and started to feel that sometimes I was losing control of myself completely. I was still trying to do without Ativan which was not helping and it took another trip to the doctor's to make me come to my senses and take them regularly again. They definitely helped me a little, making me feel more positive, but I still did not feel well and I kept thinking that one day I would wake up out of the nightmare and be like a normal person again. Throughout this time I still clung on to the dream that when I found happiness I would be fine.

As 1986 was coming to a close I was eager to finish the extension I was working on so that I could start the New Year with the pressure of work off. It was a close thing but I managed and a little reluctantly cleared the site. I say reluctantly because when I left I would be losing my last contact with Karen and all hope along with it. Nevertheless, I resigned myself to the fact that I had lost Karen and quietly in my mind I said goodbye to her.

I spent Christmas with the family in Norfolk, returning to Bagshot in the New Year, back to a lonely house without even Charlie to keep me company. It was the first time that I wondered if I could go on much longer; the feelings of isolation and loneliness were particularly strong at that time. Somehow I kept going by preparing plans for the kitchen extension and having a regular drink in the evenings. Drink was a big help to me still, because it helped me to relax and take my mind off my problems. I had found a suitable pub, called the Plough, which was situated at the other end of the town, and it was not long before I was accepted as 'part of the furniture' in the evenings.

At this time I was very well aware that I had to keep a fair amount of self-discipline, otherwise I was sure that I would lose control completely. I, therefore, made certain rules for myself to abide by and stick to them no matter what. These included restricting my drinking from nine o'clock in the evening only. I was determined to keep a certain routine in my life.

Being on a regular dose of Ativan was a problem to me because I knew eventually I would get used to it and it would lose its therapeutic value, so once again I decided to take it only when it was absolutely essential. Doing this meant my life would be harder, but I thought there was no other real alternative.

There was a lot of confusion in my head about why I felt like I did, but the one thought that became more and more prominent was the feeling that I had been taken over by something evil and it was out to destroy me. With this in mind I contacted a Spiritualist friend and had a chat, but it was not very fruitful because she said she could not sense anything wrong at all. Nevertheless, I remained convinced and decided that maybe the evil could be undetectable.

With so much going on in my head it took all the strength I had left to concentrate on starting the kitchen extension that I had been given the go ahead to do. Right from the start every shovel full of earth, every brick laid and every piece of timber sawn was stressful to me. But however bad I felt I was determined, more than ever, to see the project through to completion.

Halfway through the extension I started to run out of money. Somehow I had miscalculated the amount needed and as my Income Support only covered day to day expenses I had no option but to sell my precious car. It turned out a lot harder to sell than it was to buy and in the end I lost a lot of money on it. I still needed transport, so I purchased an old banger which would have to do until I sold the house.

Now I had the money I needed I decided there was no rush to finish the work, although I still had to be careful not to spend too much on drink. It was very tempting to buy drinks for different people when down the pub and I often had to discipline myself against 'a could not care less' attitude that I often had.

The Plough became my second home and it was there that I met up with a familiar face. Her name was Samantha and she used to be a barmaid at my old drinking hole, the Fox and Hounds. I had always fancied her but the fact that she was married put me off, until now! In conversation she told me she had split with her husband recently and was slowly coming to terms with it. When she was about to leave we exchanged phone numbers and she said she would ring me.

For days I waited for Sam to call me but she did not and, although painful for me I did not ring her either. It was about three weeks before she came into the pub again and when she did she greeted me with a smile. It was then that all my hidden emotions came to the surface and I was helpless to stop them. In what I can only describe as an emotional frenzy I blurted out that I was sorry I had not rung and that I missed her. Her reaction was one of sheer horror and disbelief, and I knew that I had blown it yet again. When I arrived home I vented my anger on myself and cursed myself at the top of my voice. The ranting and raving carried on for about half an hour before I burst into tears, eventually falling into a fitful sleep.

Things did not improve after that and on subsequent visits to the pub it was plain that I had lost any respect that I originally had. Matters eventually came to a head one evening when I overheard some people taking the Mickey out of me. It played on my mind all evening and as closing time approached I started an argument with a female member of staff and I was consequently asked to leave and never return. On arriving home I felt hurt and bewildered and rather annoyed because of all the money I had spent in the pub and also, although petty, the argument was in my favour!

By that time I had become very disillusioned with my life and felt very lonely. All my friends seemed to have gone out of my life and all my ten years in Surrey were virtually fruitless, so all I really had left was my house and the money it represented. I felt feeble and unwanted. I started using another pub in Bagshot after that and decided that I would keep myself to myself, because I did not need anyone else and that is the way I wanted it!

I had plenty of time to think and make plans while I worked to complete my extension; although my stress level remained high I managed to make two important decisions. Firstly I would sell my house in Bagshot as soon as possible and move up to Norfolk. Secondly, I would go abroad again to hopefully start a new life and prove to myself that I can be happy, and once I was established, wherever I went, I would move my assets along with me.

By the summer of 1987 I had finished all the work on my house and was ready to put it on the market. My plans had altered slightly by then and I had a very exciting idea that had slowly developed in my mind. It had been triggered by a video I had seen called 'The Jazz Singer', and I had been profoundly moved by a certain scene in the film. I was so profoundly moved that I strongly believed that it was a sign from God showing me where to go. Similar things had been meaningful to me, including the silent phone calls, which incidentally had carried on even though I had moved, but this scene had the biggest impact to date and I felt that I could not ignore it.

The film was about a Jewish singer who made it to the big time in Los Angeles, and Neil Diamond played the lead. He sang a number of hit songs in the film including 'Hello Again', which was played when he returned to Los Angeles after being away for some time, finding his partner on the beach with their new-born baby. The moment when she sensed that he was there was particularly moving and somehow I associated the scene with me.

My mind was made up I would go to Los Angeles and find my destiny. As soon as I had made up my mind I had to share it with someone, so I rang up Mum and told her. She was pleased that I was moving to Norfolk, but was not too impressed about Los Angeles.

Once again I sold my property pretty quickly. I was not surprised because the finished extension fitted in well. I wasted no time, and sold all my furniture, just leaving my clothes and the smaller items which I put into boxes ready to transport to Norfolk. I had already arranged with Mum and Tom to stay with them until my trip to America, so everything was going like clockwork. The day to move came in the middle of August and, with all my worldly goods squeezed into the car, I said a quiet goodbye to Surrey and set off. The trip to Norfolk proved to very unpleasant and stressful. Everything was fine until I reached the M25, but as soon as I was on it my old fear when driving came back with vengeance! As the cars on the motorway overtook me I started to feel nervous and afraid that I would lose control of the car. It was the worst that I had ever felt and I became so tense that I felt I could not even steer the car properly. The inevitable happened, I had a panic attack and I knew it was imperative that I left the motorway at the next exit, and with this in mind I stayed in the inside lane. I also knew that if I stopped on the hard shoulder I would feel just as vulnerable, if not more so. I kept saying to myself, 'concentrate, concentrate', over and over again and every time I was not surrounded by traffic I accelerated, and five minutes seemed like an hour!

The exit road was just a little further and all my concentration was focused on making it to that slip road. I kept all my emotions in check until I finally reached the exit and turned into a normal road before stopping beside an entrance to a field. I must have sat there for a good twenty minutes trying to rationalise my thoughts and chain smoking, wondering what to do next. I took a couple of Ativan and got out of the car to find I was shaking right down to my shoes. I did my best to walk a few yards, trying to loosen my tight muscles and smoked another cigarette.

Eventually I relaxed enough to sit back in the car and think about the rest of the journey. When I felt ready I started the car and turned round and drove back on to the motorway.

It was good to be back with the family again even if it was just for a short while. Mum eagerly looked for suitable properties for me, while I finalised my plans for my trip to America. We eventually found a new house in Norwich that suited my requirements so without wasting any time I enlisted the help of a solicitor whose first job was to give Mum 'power of attorney' while I was out of the country.

There was plenty to do and this was good for me as it gave me no time to think of my problems. On top of all that I still firmly believed that going away this time would sort me out for good. I intended to do as much homework on Los Angeles as possible so while I was in

London, obtaining a visa, I went to a specialist bookshop and bought various maps and books on the city. The information I obtained from the items proved invaluable. I learnt where the 'no-go' areas were, where the airport was and also that there was an area of the city, called Santa Monica, where most of the tourists stayed.

Once I had my visa there was nothing stopping me, so I obtained an air ticket at the cheapest rate possible and also rang a reasonable hotel in Santa Monica and booked to stay two weeks, which would hopefully give me time to look at alternatives. Sister Sue had a friend who knew a couple living in Los Angeles who, she seemed certain, would help me as much as possible, for which, I was very grateful. The final thing I did was to get as much Ativan from my doctor as possible.

As the big day loomed I became more and more excited even though Mum was not as enthusiastic, although she never told me so. When at last the day of departure came and I arrived at Gatwick Airport I felt a mixture of excitement and apprehension. But once again I was determined to tackle anything that life threw at me. It was just as well.

The flight was delayed five hours. Instead of taking off at eleven it was four thirty in the afternoon before the plane, a DC10, was in the air. I started my trip as I meant to go on and I took Ativan regularly, thus remaining fairly composed.

The journey, unfortunately, was in two stages. The first leg was to Houston, so I wondered when it would be that I went to bed next. I had a good few beers in the first couple of hours of the flight, and when I was suitably tanked up I tried to sleep a little. I soon found out that I was too excited to sleep so I carried on drinking and watched the in-flight movie, but the time dragged and the ten and a half hour flight seemed never ending.

On arrival at Houston I went through customs without any hassle, but it took over two hours to be told what was happening. Firstly, I waited with the rest of the passengers at baggage claim only to be told that our baggage was being kept in transit. Secondly, it took the rest of the time to be told that it was too late for a connecting flight that evening. We were given free meal vouchers and were put up in the airport hotel for the night.

In the morning there was just enough time to have a quick breakfast before boarding the connecting flight to Los Angeles. The flight took four hours and it was eleven thirty when the plane touched down. After baggage claim I took a taxi to my hotel otherwise I would have spent the rest of the day searching for it. I booked in and after settling in my room I went for a walk round the local area to try and familiarise myself with Santa Monica.

It was very hot so I did not walk too far, but did explore the beach area. The Pacific Ocean looked formidable but inviting and there were plenty of people taking advantage of the sunshine. It was typical California that I had seen on TV and there were many people jogging or roller-skating along the sea front. I made my way on to the pier and walked the whole length of it noticing the various shops, bars and restaurants as I passed by. One pub caught my eye, it was called the Crown and Anchor, and feeling I could do with a drink I went in. I was delighted to find it sold draught beer and I promptly ordered a large glass and sat at the bar to drink it.

The bartender was very attractive and as I spoke to

her I fell for her straight away. Her name was Helen and she was small with short, dark hair and a lovely smile, and during our conversation I found out she was married but was having problems because her husband was a drug addict. When I had finished my drink I decided to leave and head back to my hotel so I said goodbye to Helen, promising to return, and made my way off the pier. It was early evening when I arrived back at the hotel and I felt very tired, recognising that I had jet-lag. I was determined, however, not to sleep before bedtime so I went out again to look for something to eat after which I returned to the Crown and Anchor to finish off the day, deciding to adopt it as my local.

Up until then I had not felt too bad, I was used to a lot of symptoms so I had learned to live with them, but as the excitement of being in Los Angeles started to wear off the more troubling symptoms started to come back. Anxiety and depression were prominent and the overwhelming feeling that something was wrong haunted me. I searched my mind for the answer, covering the same ground as I had done previously. I was well aware, and worried that, it was becoming an obsession but I had to find an answer somewhere, somehow.

For the first few days I stayed close to the hotel, restricting myself to the beach and visiting the pub. Seeing Helen was the highlight of every day and I made sure she told me what shift she was on in advance. I waited until the weekend to play my trump card which was ringing up the couple whose name I had been given as a contact before I left England. The weekend came and on the Saturday I rang the number, anxious that I might not be welcome. I got through and after a short chat to both of them, Peter and Connie, they invited me to supper on the Sunday evening. They seemed all right to talk to and they gave me instructions about how to get to their home, even which bus to catch, so I was very optimistic and celebrated by getting drunk on the Saturday evening.

On the Sunday it was a very hot day. I caught the bus as instructed and alighted in the centre of Hollywood. Peter and Connie lived in the Hollywood Hills and buses did not call there so Peter had said that he would pick me up. He arrived on time and took me on the short journey to his home and on arrival I could not help but be impressed with his house and the view from it.

Peter and Connie were, I guessed, about forty and had a young daughter about ten. They made me feel welcome, but stopped short of making me feel at ease - although at this time I never really felt at ease. I was sure that they considered me a burden that they could well do without. However, during supper we discussed my plans and Peter, whom I found out was involved with show business, told me to be patient about finding work but maybe he could help. He also gave me the phone number of a girl who had accommodation and suggested I ring her at the earliest possible moment.

On arrival back in Santa Monica it was fairly late so I decided to have an early night. I did not sleep well because my mind was so active, but it did give me time to reflect on the last few days and assess my mental state. Although I was not feeling too bad I still putting up with the usual amount of stress, but by now I was used to that. The main thing, I decided, was to keep optimistic and not to let the awful depression take hold again.

Keeping up the momentum the next day I phoned

the number Peter had given me and spoke to the girl, called Anna, who I later found out, was Swedish. After a brief chat she agreed to pick me up and take me to see the house and meet her friends. With gratitude I met her and was taken a few miles across L.A. to a valley the other side of Hollywood Hills. On arrival Anna introduced me to her friends, who were also Swedish. I found out that three of them shared the house, but they had room for me if I was interested. I said that I was interested but needed a car before I could move in, so with the help of Anna we scoured the papers.

We went to see two cars that afternoon without success, but rang up a young woman who said she needed her car for a little while longer and that she would ring me at my hotel when she had bought another. It sounded promising so I decided to wait for her call and meanwhile try to cement a relationship with Anna and the others.

Anna continued to act as my taxi and ferried me to and from the house every day. I helped out with the petrol, but after a couple of days our relationship showed a bit of strain, so I thought it best if I stayed in Santa Monica until I had transport.

It was still very hot and for the next couple of days I went on the beach and visited different bars. By then I was quite familiar with the local area and soon got to know where it was safe to go, especially at night. My regular haunt at night was still the Crown and Anchor and it was inevitable that I met the owner. His name was Tommy and he originally came from Scotland, although he told me he had been in L.A. for twelve years. As the evenings passed I got to know and like Tommy and I learnt what an easy going guy he was, and soon realised he had money.

It was the morning of October 2nd 1987 and I had just woken up and was watching TV in my hotel room when at approximately a quarter to eight I feared for my life. Before then I had only read about it or seen it in films, but now it was really happening and I was in the middle of it, an Earthquake!

My room started shaking violently, and recognising what it was I leapt out of bed, grabbed my jeans and dashed out of the door and down the stairs into the street below. As I watched I could see the surrounding buildings vibrating, and looking down the skyline saw the big tower blocks swaying back and forth.

It was a terrifying experience and I just stood there with, by now a crowd of people, and watched transfixed on what was happening around us. It must have lasted a good thirty seconds, but seemed much longer and even when all was quiet nobody moved for at least another half minute.

It took me a long time to recover, and to gain enough confidence to return to my room to quickly dress so I could head for the comparative safety of the beach. I remained there for a couple of hours while everyday life returned back to something like normality. Everywhere I went for the rest of the day the talk was about the earthquake, and I found it increasingly hard to relax and get it out of my mind. I was glad to see the day out and come the evening I went and got drunk at the Crown and Anchor.

Some good news came the following day. I arrived back at the hotel at lunch time to find a message waiting for me. The young lady with the car had phoned saying that the car was ready, so without further ado I called her back and arranged to go round and see it that afternoon.

It was only a short bus ride away and I found the address easily, to be greeted by the very attractive young lady! The car was a bargain and only cost me fifty dollars which I handed over gratefully, and in return I received the keys to my freedom of travelling the highways of L.A.

Before I left with the car I was offered a cup of coffee, which I accepted, and it was after that I realised I had to ask my host out on a date. Of course, with this intention I started to tense up and became very nervous and by the time I finally asked her I was a gibbering wreck. She was very nice in refusing and made the excuse that she was recuperating from an illness, but I knew it was another lost cause so I left hastily to hide my embarrassment.

The next few days I had to get used to living with the three Swedish people. In this time I quickly realised that I was not going to be accepted as one of them, there were various reasons for this. Firstly, they continued to speak in Swedish together even in my company.

Secondly, they did not try to speak to me at all except when I spoke to them and most of them talked about me behind my back thinking that I could not hear or understand! The only good thing to come from my new found friends was that I learnt that Anna had an American friend who was small, dark and had tiny feet, and was apparently psychic! I knew if it was the last thing I did I had to meet this lady.

About a week into living in the house I started to feel down. I realised that I had to do something fast to change my fortune otherwise I would once again slip into depression and that would mean disaster. To compound my problems I was getting short of money, so I needed work and soon. I rang Peter and Connie who understood my predicament and said I could have a day shifting wood round theirs if I wanted. I accepted their kind offer and the following day went over and did the work.

It was a long hot day and by the end of it I was completely worn out. I had not enjoyed the work at all and unfortunately it only reinforced my growing disillusionment. I was paid a mere thirty-five dollars for my time which, I reflected, was all I felt I was worth. I felt like crying, but did not, instead I drove to Santa Monica and had a drink in the Crown and Anchor. I had more to drink than I should have, and drove home, which was silly because if I had been caught I would have been slung in jail. I made it home safely.

In the early hours of the morning there was an after shock from the earthquake which shook the whole house. I did not leave my bed as I was starting to not give a damn. When I did get up the house was empty, so I decided to stay in and think about what to do next.

While I sat deep in thought the phone rang. I answered it to find it was Anna's American friend. I told her Anna was not in but said that I had heard a lot about her and could I meet her in the evening. To my surprise she said she would, so we arranged a time and place and told her that I would look forward to our meeting. The rest of my day was spent in anticipation and wondering how the evening would go.

She was very small and quite attractive, but was older than I had imagined, about forty. I knew she was not my 'little lady' straight away, but as we chatted I found that she was very easy to talk to. Very soon I was pouring my heart out to her and telling her all my problems, especially about how depressed I felt. I learnt that she too had suffered from depression and had sought professional help and consequently was now much better. She urged me to return home and do the same. Again, that night I did a lot of thinking and decided that the following day I would seek help from one of the many Psychics in L.A., as I felt more than ever that my problems were spiritual.

After getting up early I made myself breakfast and then purchased a showbiz paper that I knew had lots of advertisements in. I then sat down and studied the relevant page and ringed all the possible Psychics before deciding on which one to go and see. When I had decided I rang up to arrange a time that I could go and receive a Tarot reading. To my delight I managed to get an appointment that afternoon and it would cost twenty-five dollars, which I could just afford. With great anticipation I arrived in good time to find it was quite a large shop in a busy street near the centre of the town. When I went in I was shown to a waiting area by a middle-aged woman and was told that I would not have to wait very long. After about 5 minutes a young lady about thirty came in and asked me to follow her into a dimly lit room at the rear of the shop. We then sat down at a small table where she produced a pack of Tarot cards. I then shuffled them as she asked and handed her seven cards from the pack which she took and laid face down on the table. She then proceeded to tell me a little about myself, which, I found was fairly accurate, before she suddenly went all serious and said she had discovered something that was not very nice.

Apparently there had been someone in my past that had been upset by something that had been done to them and this person had blamed my family and ultimately put a curse on me as punishment. On hearing this, instead of being appalled I was somewhat relieved because at last I had found the reason for all my problems. The suspicions I had held for the last couple of years turned out to be true! It also dawned on me that my decision to come to L.A. had been absolutely right and I had found my destiny at last!

As I sat there trying to compose myself the psychic said that she could help me get rid of the curse but it involved using nine candles. With this news I felt even more elated, realising that all the suffering and hardship that had occurred and was still occurring in my life would very soon be over. Of course, by then, I was already impatient to get it over with but knew, without asking that it would cost money and money was what I was very short of.

With trepidation I asked how much the cure would cost and was told that each candle cost twenty-five dollars, so in total it came to two hundred and twenty-five dollars. Thinking it was a lot of money, but knowing that it would be worth every penny I left the shop promising to return as soon as I could raise the cash. Late that night I rang Mum, and full of excitement told her about the day's happenings and asked her to send me two hundred pounds as soon as possible. Mum did not seem to share my excitement but agreed to send the money, so I was grateful to her and told her so. We chatted for a very short while, but learned there had been a hurricane in England, so although I had experienced an earthquake I had missed out on the hurricane!

My relationship with my Swedish housemates was deteriorating all the time and things came to a head one night when I was locked out and unable to find a key that was supposed to be left for me. Feeling frustrated and angry I discovered an open window which I managed to get through, but in doing so I broke the blind on the inside. When the others returned they were not too happy with me and after a short debate it was decided I would go as soon as possible.

As I lay in my bunk that night, unable to sleep, I realised that I had to find somewhere to live and fast. I was not particularly bothered because I knew my luck would change as soon as the money arrived and the curse was removed. I was half asleep when I suddenly remembered a phone number I had been given. It was the number of an English couple I had met in the Crown and Anchor during the first week after I arrived in L.A. I searched through my wallet and found it and decided to ring them in the morning.

It was the lady who answered the phone when I rang, and on hearing her voice I recalled that they were a very nice couple. Her name was Sandy and his was Ray. She remembered me and seemed pleased that I had rung and invited me over to see them in their electrical shop with perhaps dinner afterwards. They worked and lived in Sun Valley which was the other side of L.A., but I had no trouble finding them and arrived at their shop in the mid-morning.

Both Sandy and Ray made me feel welcome, which was a refreshing change, and it was not very long before I was talking freely to them. They soon learnt that I was short of money and needed work desperately, so with this news Sandy picked up the phone and rang her friend who ran a sister shop in a place called Lancaster which was about twenty miles away in the desert. Her friend told Sandy that she wanted part of her shop painted and would I like to go and see her, so, of course, I said 'Yes'.

Before I left for Lancaster, Sandy and Ray bought me a sandwich and kindly gave me five dollars to cover petrol for my journey. As I set off I felt really touched by the kindness they had shown me and even shed a couple of tears. As I thought more about them I prayed that the curse that was on me would not upset our new friendship. It made me even more determined that I would do everything within my power to alleviate the problem as soon as possible.

Lancaster was a new town, but still had the characteristic main street with similar roads branching off it. The shop was at the far end of the town on the main street, so I found it quite quickly. They were expecting me and once again I found a warm reception. They showed me the work to be done and said I could start the next day if I wanted and, of course, I agreed especially after they said I would be paid one hundred and seventy dollars for my efforts.

On arriving home in the early evening I told Anna that I would pay some rent in a couple of days which seemed to please her. I still needed a roof over my head for a little while longer. I decided to have an early night, so I retired to bed soon after ten o'clock, especially as the conversation in the house was again so riveting. Many thoughts went round in my head that night and again I found sleep hard to come by. I was now very determined not to be beaten and give in to the curse that was upon me.

In the morning I made my way over to Sun Valley, again to be warmly greeted by Ray and Sandy. I went with Sandy to get the paint, brushes and other things, and before I left for Lancaster Sandy gave me 10 dollars and wished me luck. Once again I thought about the kindness of Ray and Sandy and hoped that one day I would be in a position to return it.

I made it to Lancaster by mid-day and after a

sandwich for lunch started work. It was six o'clock when the shop closed and I finished work for the day. I had got on well and was pretty sure I would finish it the next day. As it was not worth returning home and I had noticed a cheap Motel along the highway, I decided to book in there for the night. Considering the price, my room was not too bad and it even had a shower which I made full use of. Afterwards, feeling refreshed, I discovered a burger bar up the road so I ate there before making my way over to the Holiday Inn where I spent the remains of my money getting drunk!

It was a pleasant evening, mainly because there was an excellent group performing in the bar and by the time they finished I was more than ready for bed. As I made my way unsteadily back to the Motel I was walking by the side of the road when a pair of car headlights came towards me and I was completely dazzled.

The car stopped in front of me and out jumped the two occupants, a man and a woman, they were police officers. Just like in the movies I was told to freeze, so I stood as still as I could while the policeman searched me for weapons. After, of course, finding nothing he told me to empty my pockets and when he saw that I did not have any money he became suspicious and asked me where the drugs were. At this point I noticed his attitude left a lot to be desired, but without reacting I told him I was drunk not on drugs, but I could see that he did not believe me.

When asked, I told the two officers where I was staying, so they drove to my Motel (with me in the back of the car) and searched my room and my car. The policeman still seemed reluctant to believe I was clean and I did not really want to disclose too much because I was, after all, working illegally. Eventually, after a discussion amongst themselves, they left and I went to bed.

The following day went slowly, the main reason for that was because I could not seem to focus my mind and concentrate. The only way I can describe it is that my mind was full of rubbish, with different, irrelevant and unnecessary thoughts going round and round in my head. It was a real toil to finish the painting, but somehow I soldiered on and when I had completed the task and I was driving home I nearly fell asleep at the wheel, I was very tired.

After the usual welcome back at the house I went straight to bed. Having no reason to stay at home, the next day I spent in Santa Monica mostly trying to relax my mind on the beach. I took an extra Ativan to help me but I knew I had to see my Psychic friend and get the curse lifted; otherwise I would go completely barmy. The money I asked Mum to send had not arrived yet, which reinforced my fear that the curse was influencing matters and it was becoming a competition between me and it. I had to stay strong and not be beaten, because I wanted my life back and that to me was the biggest incentive of all!

That evening I went in the Crown and Anchor hoping upon hope to see little Helen. I wanted to tell her what I was going through, I wanted to tell her everything, I wanted her to love me, but she was not working. While I sat at the bar I got talking to a big guy with a beard who I later found out was an ex-Hell's Angel. He was a nice man and after a couple of drinks we went to various other bars in Santa Monica. One bar in particular I liked was called Annie's, I liked it mainly because of the young girl bartender who was very sexy and knew it, and I was very turned on by her! As the evening progressed and drink followed drink I made it obvious what I thought of her and seemed to get a positive reaction back, but by then I was drunk and incapable so I left saying I would return. I slept in the car that night!

The depression I feared started to return and for the next couple of days I tried to keep busy. Sandy and Ray were once again good to me, buying me lunch and petrol, but they did not have any further work for me. Despondency started to take hold but I was still determined to beat it and with that attitude I had my first big break!

I was in the Crown and Anchor talking to Helen when a friend of hers walked in. She introduced him as Chuck and as far as I could make out he was about my age. We soon became engrossed in conversation; mainly because he was so easy going and I learnt that he was in the construction trade. All evening we talked and I began to like Chuck and I still believe today that if circumstances had been different we would have become great mates. As we left the bar he promised to keep in touch and told me to be patient about work because he had many contacts. I drove home that night and realised how silly it was, because again I knew had I been caught I would have been put in jail!

The Crown and Anchor continued to be my favourite haunt as I had met the majority of my contacts there. It was there that I again met my ex-biker friend who liked to be known as Bear. Bear was formidable to look at and I guessed in his younger days was even more formidable. In a very short time I grew to like him and this particular night I had reason to. We had been in the pub all night and shortly before leaving he said that he have managed to find me a couple of days work detailing cars. Now, at first I was not impressed as I did not like the idea of cleaning cars all day, but as he explained he owed the proprietor a favour and I would be doing him a great service. I could not refuse, as I owed Bear a lot in drinks and loans. When I accepted, he said in that case I could stay round his for the night. Detailing was very hard work and I was not even allowed to smoke, but the time went relatively quickly and at the end of the two days I picked up 70 dollars!

With the money in my pocket I returned to the house and decided to have a night in. While half watching television I picked up a newspaper and read the small ads. I came across a section asking for film extras and thought, why not!

In the morning I rang an agency and made an appointment for the afternoon. When I went along, they said I would have to pay 30 dollar's induction fee but I was guaranteed at lest one job. I paid the money and was told to report to a night club the following day.

It was a long day, but very interesting. It was a low budget film with unknown actors called 'Johnny Guitar' and as the day progressed I managed to get into quite a few shots! I also managed to get to know a girl who was very friendly and loved my English accent. As the day drew to a close I offered to take her home. She said 'Yes', if her parents did not mind, so I rang them but they were already on their way to pick her up. I was so frustrated that I told her to piss off, which I regretted but by then it was too late. Once again I had missed out and I wondered if I would ever have sex again, as I could not remember the last time!

That evening at the Crown and Anchor I began to think about the curse again. It was stopping me getting on in L.A. I knew I had to stay strong and never give in to it and prayed that the money from home would arrive soon. It was as if the curse was affecting me receiving and earning enough money to get it lifted.

Caught up in my thoughts I did not see Chuck come into the pub and it was only when a drink was put in front of me that I noticed his big grin. We sat and chatted with Helen for a while. She was as lovely as ever and when we had finished our drinks Chuck told me to follow him as he had a surprise for me. We walked further up the pier until we reached the amusement stalls, where we entered a small office. Once in the office, Chuck introduced me to Kirk who he said was a good friend of his. Kirk was a guy of about fifty who was an ex New York cop, but in spite of that seemed very nice. He asked a few questions and seeming satisfied said I could start on one of the stalls the next day if I wished. I thanked him and said I would but would he pay me cash? He replied that cash would not be a problem and I would get 3 dollars 50 cents an hour. Chuck and I returned to the Crown and Anchor where I celebrated by buying us a drink. When Chuck left I thanked him again and turned my attention, yet again to Helen. Although she had turned me down before I thought I would try once again to get her to go out with me. My efforts were, once again, in vain. Feeling rebuked I finished my drink quickly and went home.

The next couple of days being the weekend I started working on the amusement stall. My stall was the 'Get the ball in the milk churn', which proved to be very boring. My workmates were mostly Mexicans, but all spoke good English and seemed fairly friendly. As it was out of season the amusements were only open at weekends, so I had to look for other work for week days.

On the Monday I received a big boost. The money from home arrived at the house and at first I could not believe my eyes. When it finally sank in I felt elated and suddenly very nervous, knowing that at last I had the means to lift the curse that had been plaguing me for so long. As I sat contemplating and looking at the phone number I had kept in my wallet, I felt a great urgency to ring the number and get things over and done with.

There was no reply, which was frustrating to say the least. By then I was coiled up like a spring and needed satisfaction straight away. I felt desperate and rushed upstairs to retrieve the paper with all the advertisements in. I scanned the pages, eventually coming across a prominent ad that bore the name Gina. I picked up the phone once again and rang the new number. It was answered almost immediately by a girl, who introduced herself as Carrie.

Carrie sounded a very nice girl and I warmed towards her immediately. I did not tell her about my problems but arranged an appointment for a Tarot reading in the afternoon. After lunch I got into my car and made my way over to see Carrie. It was about fifteen miles to the San Fernando Valley where she lived and my excitement made it seem a lot further.

Eventually I arrived for my reading and the front door was opened by a girl of about twenty wearing what I can only describe as a white gown. She introduced herself as Carrie and, hardly making a sound as she walked, showed me to an armchair where she asked me to sit down. She sat opposite me and produced pack of Tarot cards and put them in front of me. As the reading progressed I became less impressed with my host because she was not telling me what I wanted to hear. Finally, before she finished talking I started telling her about the previous Psychic I had seen and about the curse and how desperate I was to get it lifted. After a short time of meditation she collected together all the cards and asked me to shuffle them and pick out three. This I did and she laid them in front of her, and suddenly became very serious. She then started to relate to me what she saw and said that there was indeed a curse on me and that it had been around for several years. I asked her if she could do anything about it and she replied by saying that with plenty of meditation she could, but it take a bit of time and money. I gave her 50 dollars to get on with and left feeling frustrated that I had to wait still more days before I was free, although Carrie did say that things should improve as she worked.

The following two days I worked at Peter and Connie's doing little odd jobs around their property. This helped to take my mind off the curse for a few hours, however as Carrie told me, things should improve with time I was constantly searching for signs of improvement. They were warm days and it was very peaceful up in the hills and it soon triggered off emotions that I had not felt for a long time, although they were somewhat jumbled. I felt very emotional as an intense feeling of peace nearly overwhelmed me, but as it faded I tried desperately to hang onto it because for those few moments in time I felt very close to God.

I rang Carrie that evening to tell her how I had felt and she was pleased because she said she had been working very hard for me. After the phone call I became very emotional again realising that at last things were improving and every day I should get better and better with Carrie's help. At that moment in time money did not matter to me as I would gladly have given Carrie everything as long as eventually I had my life back!

Matters stood still towards the weekend and I felt no further improvement in myself. Friday was a bad day. Firstly, I had a puncture in the morning which meant buying a new tyre and, low and behold, I had another blow-out in the afternoon. So, that day I had to purchase two new tyres which came to over 60 dollars! To finish the day off I had a heart to heart with my Swedish housemates which eventually ended in me saying I would move out Sunday evening. That gave me two days to find another room or digs otherwise I would have to sleep in the car. In the evening I rang Carrie and told her about my misfortune which resulted in her telling me that it was the curse fighting back, but I was not to worry because it was getting weaker all the time. My feelings were muddled by Saturday, on one side there was Carrie working hard for me to lift the curse and on the other I was cutting down my intake of Ativan because firstly, my supply was getting low and secondly, I believed in what Carrie was doing - so therefore I should not have to take so many.

    That Saturday evening I was in the Crown and Anchor after working on my stall when I began talking to a chap and his wife. We found we had a fair bit in common as he worked in the building trade and as the conversation progressed onto other things I told them I was looking for somewhere to stay. On hearing this they discussed something between themselves and seemed to come to an agreement. Turning to me, the chap asked me if I wanted to stay on his construction site which was just up the road, saying that it was dry and fenced in. In reply I asked him if it was possible to see it and he immediately agreed. The three of us left the pub and drove in his car to the site. It was situated in a fairly quiet area of Santa Monica, close to the sea, and as the couple unlocked the gate of the compound I noticed two site huts inside. Reading my mind, the chap said I could not sleep in the huts because there was a lot of valuable equipment in them but I could sleep anywhere within the half finished building they were constructing.

With my mind made up I surveyed my new sleeping quarters and noticed how draughty it was, realising I would have to obtain a sleeping bag. I was given the keys to the compound and driven back to the pub where I said goodbye to the couple and jumped into my car and went back to the house to spend my last night in relative comfort. In the morning, before I left to go to work, I rang Sandy and Ray in Sun Valley and as usual they seemed pleased to hear from me. I told them the latest news, including the fact that I was low on tablets. Sandy was particularly sympathetic and said she would make an appointment with her doctor for me, saying that she would also pay the fee. She also said that they had a sleeping bag I could borrow. Once again I became very emotional over Sandy and Ray's kindness and hoped upon hope that I would one day be able to repay them.

When I picked up the sleeping bag on Sunday evening I was invited to dinner and had a lovely cooked meal. Apart from the food it was a distressing evening for me, mainly because I felt anxious and on edge. I left soon after the meal apologising to Sandy and Ray. Sandy was concerned about me but I told her not to worry, although wishing I knew what was wrong with me.

My first night on the construction site was not the most comfortable, but I managed to find some cardboard to lie on which helped a little and eventually I had a little sleep. I prayed softly for strength because I felt so isolated and alone. The next morning I returned to Ray and Sandy's shop in Sun Valley and sat and chatted to Sandy as she worked. While I was there she rang the doctor and surprised me with an appointment the same afternoon.

The doctor was a pleasant man and did not question my need for Ativan; he just simply wrote out a prescription for a 100 and gave it to me. I paid the 40 dollar fee (which Sandy had given me) and returned to Sandy and Ray's shop, to say thanks and goodbye, before going to a large Drug Emporium to get my prescription changed. It was a relief to have a good supply of Ativan once again, but if I remember rightly I had to part with another 35 dollars to get them.

Whether it was the waiting for the curse to be lifted or whether it was the lack of money and no weekday job that was affecting me, the sad fact of the matter was I felt rough. I felt so bad that it was beginning to rub off into my behaviour. I was under the most stress I had ever been in my life. The negative fears that had been affecting me for so long were now constantly on my mind. I was becoming petrified that I would lose control of myself and even of saying the wrong thing. Every thought that came into my head I found myself analysing and vetting, so it was extremely hard to hold a conversation with anyone without losing concentration and forgetting what was being talked about. Consequently I began to avoid long conversations. In fact, I wished to be alone with my thoughts so I could work my way through them and get some rationality back, but it was very, very hard, it was like a maze.

One evening I seemed to lose heart for the fight and for an instant I thought that was it, I had succumbed to the curse and all was lost. I phoned Carrie and told her I needed her help desperately, because without it I would probably lose control of myself and end up in trouble or worse still prison or even a mental institution. She told me to wait on the phone.

The next voice I heard was authoritative and demanded respect. It was a woman's voice. The first thing she said was that her name was Gina and that she was Carrie's mother. She then told me to listen very carefully. In a slow clear voice she told me that there was not a curse on me but something a lot more serious and that it needed a lot more work. The next thing she told me came as an immense shock and stunned me speechless, although I totally believed what she said! 'You have a spirit of a dead person inside you and it is trying to take over you. You used to know this person as she was a relative of yours. It is your Grandmother, your mother's mother'.

Gina also went on to say that I must trust her to help me and not to tell anyone else, because it would make matters even worse. She finished by saying that I should come and see her the next day.

When I put the phone down a feeling of desperation came over me and I was close to panic. I knew I had to hold things together because if I did not there would be no coming back and this would be doubly serious in a foreign country. I stood next to the phone booth for a good ten minutes trying to compose myself, speaking to myself, calming myself, until slowly the panic subsided and I was able to think more rationally. As I stood there I could feel a pressure in my chest, which I knew was the spirit inside me as I could feel it moving around! I felt sick and dirty, both inside and out but I knew I would have to put up with it for a while longer. I remember saying to myself that if things were not so serious they would be funny, and raising a little smile!

The Crown and Anchor was open, so I got drunk. I met Chuck in the pub, he did his best to cheer me up and almost succeeded, but I did apologise for my behaviour. I slept in the car that night.

After an uncomfortable night I woke up abruptly with the memories of the previous night still uppermost in my mind. The pressure in my chest had subsided, but I still felt sick and unable to face food. Still in a daze I went for a cup of coffee, returning to my car as quickly as possible so that I could go over and see Gina. It was a Friday and there was a lot of traffic on the freeways (even more than usual), but I arrived at Gina's in good time. As I waited at the front door I noticed that I was thinking a bit more rationally than of late and wondered whether Gina was the reason.

Gina answered the door herself. She was a lady who at a guess was in her late forties, tidily dressed with short hair. Her one overwhelming feature was her calmness and confidence; she had a definite aura about her that said 'do not cross me' or 'cross me at your peril'. Right from the start I looked up to her and respected her and she must have known this because she was relaxed with me straight away.

Time was always precious with Gina, I found that out on our first meeting, however, she made enough time to tell me that 'the spirit' could be removed but it would take a lot of time and hard work because she would have to go through my whole life and cleanse every part that had been contaminated and the only time she could do it was at night. She then asked me if I had any money and I replied not much but I could get some sent from

England, so she told me to do so saying that she needed at least 100 dollars a week.

    Before leaving Gina I implored her to start work immediately, promising her money very shortly, to which she replied, 'ok'. In relief I asked her how long it would take and she replied about five to six weeks. On hearing this, my heart sank and I immediately wondered if I could last so long, but I knew I had no choice! I left Gina's feeling desperate and alone, so I made my way over to Sun Valley to visit Sandy and Ray knowing that I could not tell them a thing about my predicament. That night I rang Mum expecting an argument, but to my surprise she said she would send another 300 dollars. She seemed concerned about me, but I told her that very soon everything would be all right and not to worry about me. It was a short call, but long enough to make me feel homesick!

    When I settled down for the night, snuggled up in my sleeping bag on the construction site, I was aware of the pressure in my chest once again, but I tried to ignore it and said a short prayer for God to keep me safe. It was surprisingly quiet except for the odd car going past and I tried to clear my mind of all thoughts, but did not succeed so I concentrated on thinking about good things and reminisced about the girls that had touched my life, and recalled the warm emotions I had felt when with the special ones. It seemed to work, for although I became very emotional I slowly drifted off to sleep.

Money was short again so I stayed away from the Crown and Anchor except for the weekend when I worked on the stall. They were long days as I was always up at the crack of dawn, preferring to avoid the workmen as they came to work. I spent many early mornings walking along the sea front, passing many of the down and outs and Vietnam veterans that frequented the area. They soon got to recognise me and never bothered me, as if they knew I was troubled.

Thanksgiving approached, and to celebrate Sandy and Ray invited me over to their house for the customary Turkey dinner. They made it special for me because they let me shower and stay the night, making me feel more human for a couple of days. They also gave me a driving job that lasted a couple of days and paid me more than generously for doing it. The generosity Sandy and Ray showed towards me sometimes embarrassed me, as I had nothing to give in return, but they were precious friends who were always there for me.

With money in my pocket for a change I gave Gina 30 dollars and received very little comfort for it, except that I was told the work was going along nicely. Everything, however, was not going along nicely for me. I was still very stressed up and all my fears and phobias, including driving, were much in evidence. Every moment of every day was a battle and my Nana's spirit was being very troublesome.

One evening I ventured back into Annie's Bar and this time I was not with Bear. The beautiful blonde was serving again and it pleased me to know that she remembered me, greeting me with a lovely smile. As the evening progressed we started talking and for once I was fairly relaxed. The conversation somehow turned to sexual matters and the vision of loveliness in front of me complained that nowadays she had little fun because of the fear of catching Aids. I replied that we did not have that problem in England so far. Later on I was sitting at the bar when the object of my growing lust decided to sit down with her legs apart, just enough for me to catch a glance of her very white knickers. She caught me looking and smiled and it was from then that I realised that at last my luck was in!

Being relaxed, I knew would not last, but I prayed that my troublesome spirit would remain quiet and allow me a few hours of enjoyment. As I waited at the bar my stress level started to increase so I started to drink more hoping to counteract the symptoms. By the end of the night I was drunk and incapable of anything except sleep. Once again I had failed to take advantage of an opportunity of love for whatever reason, this time I knew it was not my own fault, but was down to forces of a sinister nature. Whatever the reason, however, it was still very sexually frustrating. I slept in the car that night vowing never to give up however many knocks I had to suffer, one day I would be happy!

During the days of waiting for Gina, when I had the time, I would drive up into the Hollywood Hills at night. I would find a quiet, secluded spot and look down at the lights of the city. It stretched as far as I could see, and I used to get lost in my emotions, but strangely although I was alone I never felt lonely, if anything I felt exhilarated. There was also a strong sense of being near God at this time and I knew it was a genuine feeling because God is all powerful and can override anything else. It was like therapy for me and it reinforced my will to go on with the fight.

About a week after my initial meeting with Gina I received the money from England. My early efforts to cash it failed, I must have tried every bank in Santa Monica, which piled up the frustration I felt, thinking that things were working against me again. I was finally informed that the only place to get my money changed was a place in the heart of the city.

It was late afternoon when I arrived at Gina's with the cash, but I felt relieved to get there and hand over the bulk of it. Gina was very pleased that I could finally give her a substantial sum and promised to keep working although reiterating that I should remain patient. I ate well that evening deciding to treat myself. I finished up in the Crown and Anchor where I met Bear who I actually bought a drink for, instead of the other way round.

As I lay in my sleeping bag that night on the construction site I decided that I would ring up Peter and Connie to see if they had found me anymore work. If I did not get any joy from them I would go and see Sandy and Ray and buy them lunch for once. With my morning mapped out and trying to ignore the pressure in my chest, I slept.

Peter and Connie, in complete contrast to Sandy and Ray, were not friendly towards me. They were polite and civil, but I had the impression I was an unnecessary burden for them especially as I had not hit it off with their Swedish friends. Nevertheless, when I rang them I spoke to Peter and he said he had been waiting for me to ring because he had some work for me. He told me that a neighbour of his, who was a lawyer, wanted a handyman to do odd jobs round his home. We arranged to meet him the following evening.

It was Thursday and I was looking forward to the weekend so I could work on the pier. I arrived at Peter and Connie's in the early evening, where I was offered a cup of coffee. We all sat in the garden as it was a glorious dusk and still warm enough. We chatted a little but I found it very hard to relax and I felt sure that Peter and Connie noticed, so I told them I was having a few problems but assured them that everything was under control. Peter then went on to tell me that his lawyer friend was a bit volatile, but was fine as long as you did not upset him. With this on my mind we went round to see him.

The lawyer's house was further up the hill from Peter and Connie's and much bigger, with its own swimming pool. His wife answered the door to us and with a beaming smile invited us in. We had another cup of coffee while we talked and I soon decided that although she was nice, he was not and I would have great difficulty being relaxed with him; however, as I needed the money we agreed that I would start on Monday.

The weekend passed with me working on the pier as usual and, when not working, in the Crown and Anchor. Nothing out of the ordinary happened but I still fought to hang on to my sanity as the symptoms never let up even for a minute.

When Monday came I was not looking forward to working at all, but I went and spent my first day doing different jobs around the house. My employer was away all day but his wife was there along with two nannies who I later found out were Danish. As the week progressed I started to get to know the girls fairly well and it was not long before they asked me to join them when they went out in the evening. I always declined the invitations saying that I was too busy, but on the Thursday of my first working week they asked me for the real reason why I would not go out with them. Feeling under pressure I told them that I had a few problems that I was trying to sort out and in reply they asked me what problems? I so wanted to tell them the truth, to share my burden that I finally gave in and I told them everything. It was not easy because as soon as I started the words seemed to strangle me and I felt that I was going to be sick. Despite this I carried on talking in gasps and the two girls just stood there in amazement until I explained that I should not really have told them, because I was told not to say anything about it and that was why I was very anxious when I did.

My two Danish friends were very sympathetic and understanding and totally believed my story, and told me they wished there was something they could do, but I said that it was best if they did not get involved for their own safety. That was the last I saw of them because on the Friday I fell out with the lawyer, who turned out to be very nasty and ordered me off his land, never to return!

Before I left the lawyer's property I demanded the money he owed me and after a while he conceded and gave it to me. On the way back to Santa Monica I called in to see Peter and Connie. Peter was at work, but Connie was in and she listened while I explained why I was not still working. I also apologised that it did not work out and asked her to give my apologies to Peter.

Christmas was looming on the horizon and I was feeling rotten. Since I had left the lawyer's employ I had not had any full time work. I was getting by however, doing odd jobs for Peter and Connie and also for Sandy and Ray. My mental health certainly was not getting better; in fact, I was under so much strain that communication with others was becoming increasingly difficult. My relationship with Peter and Connie all but ended at the beginning of December. I was given the task of digging up a palm tree root at their house and what I thought would be a straight forward task became a nightmare. All morning I worked and all the effort I put in was to no avail, it would not budge. While I worked I became more and more frustrated. I started getting annoyed and started to think that all I was good for was digging and carting wood around and even cleaning cars. By lunch time I had had enough and I just threw down the shovel and jumped in my car and drove over to Gina's.

Gina was in and when she opened the door I implored her to hurry up with her work so we could expel the spirit as quickly as possible. She tried to calm me down and said that it should only be a couple of more weeks. She also said that there was some work that needed doing in her new shop the following week and if I did it I would virtually pay off what I owed her. Feeling I had no choice, I agreed to do it. That evening I rang Peter and Connie and as expected they were none too pleased with me, so I just said I was sorry they felt like they did and put the phone down. I was past caring! After another evening in the Crown and Anchor I drove to the construction site and was about to bed down for the night when I noticed the site office door open. It was a lot more cosy in there, but I knew that if I was caught sleeping in there I would probably be in trouble.

Nevertheless, I trusted that I would be awake before the workmen arrived in the morning as I normally was, so I decided to take the risk. Sure enough I would have slept through but the phone saved me. It was seven o'clock the next morning when it rang and without thinking I jumped out of my sleeping bag and answered it. There was no one there, which immediately seemed familiar especially as there was about a ten second pause before disconnection. For a short while I did not realise the significance of the call until I looked at my watch and saw the time. I had just enough time to roll up my sleeping bag and straighten things out before the workmen arrived!

As I mentioned earlier, I had fallen out with Peter and Connie, who was bad enough, but there was no way I wanted to lose Sandy and Ray in the same way. But until I had got rid of the spirit that possessed me I was not confident of anything. Towards the end of my stay in America various things happened to put a strain on our relationship. The first thing was when I parked in front of their driveway and Ray reversed into my car causing a far amount of damage to his car. Another was when Ray and I went out for a drink together and I said a lot more than I should have done. Thinking back, it must have sounded weird to Ray because I kept hinting that things that happened to me that I sometimes had no control over. The last straw for Ray was when I had some photographs developed and they all seemed to be covered in blood. I did not mention blood, but Ray did not need telling, he worked it out for himself. You could see that he could not and did not want to understand what was going on. Sandy was more level headed, but was still concerned about events.

For the three remaining weeks before Christmas I tried to keep a low profile as regards to Sandy and Ray. I also became very busy towards Christmas. I was glad to be busy because it helped take my mind off things, although the obsessive thoughts the spirit created in my mind were still torturing me.

The work I did for Gina was mostly putting up shelves and hanging doors. Her new shop was quite large and had a toilet and small washroom. She had partitioned some of it off and had left her mark in various ways with velvet curtains and beaded screens and had already given it a mystical atmosphere. I found the work very hard going and things went wrong constantly. Gina said it was to be expected as the evil spirit inside me did not like working for her. I pressed on, however, and gradually got the work done but by the time I nearly had the work finished my stress level was sky high.

In the corner of Gina's shop was a statue of Christ on the Cross. It was on the floor propped up against the wall and stood about three feet high. I remember thinking how out of place it looked. As the day wore on and I had just about had enough, I was up a pair of steps when I lost my balance and had to jump clear of falling timber. I ended up in a heap on the floor, but as I fell I knocked the statue of Christ over. With my whole weight knocking against it, the statue unfortunately broke. On closer inspection I noticed that it was made of plaster and one arm was completely broken off. Gina was not amused, but said that it did not matter and picked up the pieces while I carried on working.

Two weeks before Christmas the holiday period started which meant that the amusement stalls on Santa Monica pier were open every day except Sundays. My boss, Kirk, asked me if I could work full time and I, of course, said 'Yes'. I was well pleased because I liked working on my stall and by then I had become friendly with a few of the Mexican workmates. When not busy I used to listen to the radio which was broadcast through special speakers on the stalls and I used to look forward to hearing the number one record at the time called 'No one in the World', by Anita Baker. It was a very moody song and to this day when I hear it, it takes me back to America and my time on the pier! We used to get a melting pot of various people visiting the pier, both ethnic and white people, and they were from all different classes of society, rich and poor and I even noticed a few

famous faces occasionally. The pier was always well patrolled by the police and I saw very little trouble. One particular incident I did witness was a fight between three Mexicans and a coloured guy. It happened one morning at the end of the pier and lasted about 30 seconds, in which time the coloured guy who obviously had knowledge of a martial art fought off his attackers single handed. There was quite a crowd of onlookers, but nobody went to the guy's aid, not that he needed it!
One day, nearer to Christmas, the circus came to town and set up on the car park under the pier. It had a very big reputation and from my vantage point I could see scores of people visiting the show. It was a sell out every night and judging by the number of limousines attending, frequented by the rich and famous. One night, Kirk asked a couple of us to give out leaflets advertising the pier's facilities to the visitors attending the circus. We stood at the gates by the car park and gave a leaflet to everybody that passed. Just when the show was about to start a big white stretched limousine pulled up beside us. We waited, full of anticipation, for the doors to open and when they did out jumped two very glamorous females followed by Dudley Moore!

It was just like a scene from the film 'Arthur', because Dudley Moore had obviously been drinking although he could still walk unaided. As he approached me I handed him a leaflet, which he took and read in front of me. As he went in the entrance of the circus I wished him 'Good night', and he replied 'Thanks!' That is my one main 'Claim to Fame' of my trip to the USA!

It was wonderful to have full time employment, even though it was only while the season lasted. At night, after work, I would go in the Crown and Anchor as usual and by then I regarded it as my home. The owner, Tommy, as it got nearer to Christmas started having live music in the bar which started to pull more customers in. One evening I went into the bar and ordered a drink and sat trying to relax and listened to the music. As I surveyed my surroundings I noticed a blonde, a very pretty woman about 40 sitting looking at me. At first I did not really take much notice because as usual I was preoccupied by a jungle of thoughts, but as I slowly came round I began to feel interested in her because every time I looked at her she was looking at me and smiling. Halfway through my next drink I plucked up the courage and asked her if she wanted to dance, knowing that if I missed the opportunity I would never forgive myself. She accepted my invitation and took my hand and led me to the dance area. She seemed to have a permanent smile on her face, which remained even when dancing. I was with her all evening and as every minute passed we became more and more intimate and danced to every slow tune the band played, which started to get extremely embarrassing because the way her body moved and the feel of it really turned me on.

Towards the end of the evening I had had enough of dancing and drinking and just wanted to take my passionate partner home and give her what she so obviously wanted! There was one small problem that had to be sorted out before I could have my long awaited night of love, her friend. She had sat with us the whole of the evening, occasionally getting up to dance. When I said I wanted to leave, the friend said that she would get her car and pick us up at the entrance to the pub. Neither of them objected when I got into the car, sitting in the back with my new lover. As soon as we pulled away from the pub we could not keep our hands to ourselves, we just kissed and groped each other, oblivious to anything going on around us. She certainly was a very hot lady but did something I had not encountered before, she purred like a cat when at the height of passion. I was at the stage when I could not care less what she did and although I thought purring unusual, it did not deter me.

The friend drove us to an all night restaurant where we had some coffee before driving us back near the pier, beside a block of flats which was were they lived. We all went into the building and caught the lift up to about the fifth floor where we said goodbye to the friend and the two of us walked further along a corridor before we stopped outside a flat door. My partner unlocked the door and invited me in. What happened next was, at the time beyond belief! As I approached my hostess with arms outstretched, she backed away with a look of sheer panic on her face. No amount of coaxing or persuasion on my pat would get her to calm down and in the end she opened the door again and more or less begged me to leave. By this time I was very bemused and very frustrated, so without hesitation and in full view of my frightened friend got on her bed and removed my trousers and underwear and masturbated.

Later, as I lay in my sleeping bag I still could not believe what had happened earlier that night. I had left the flat quickly because I had remembered my car was parked on a tow away zone. As I went to leave, the woman suddenly changed her mind again and more or less begged me not to go. I walked out of the flat and into the corridor as she grabbed my arm and pleaded with me not to go, meanwhile I was literally dragging her along the shiny floor. In the end she let go of me and returned to her flat in some distress.

The following day I rang Gina and asked her how much longer I would have to suffer the misfortunes I was experiencing. She told me that she had nearly finished the cleansing and to ring her the following day. That evening I went into the Crown and Anchor and sat with Tommy, who immediately asked me how I had fared the previous evening. I told him and he laughed, saying that he should have told me before but did not because he thought that I would realise it myself. In answer I said, 'Realise what!' Then he said that the woman in question suffered from Schizophrenia!

I had encountered Schizophrenia before and remembered how sorry I felt for the person involved. I felt the same way this time and wished that there was something I could do to help the poor girl, but knew that interference would not be wise. All I knew at that moment was that some other people's problems made mine seem minuscule in comparison, and at least my problems would be sorted out very soon.

Sleep was a problem that night, mainly because I was excited about the fact that very soon I would be free and be my own person again. I wanted to ring Gina there and then but knew that I had to wait until the morning. As I lay there in my sleeping bag on the construction site everything seemed quiet and peaceful, and even the pressure in my chest had subsided as though the spirit was resigned to defeat. I slept eventually.

Gina gave me instructions when I rang, telling me that it was necessary to collect some leaves and earth from the ground and rub them all over my body twice a day for two days, and to ring her again at the end of the period. I felt a bit foolish at first, because everywhere I tried to do it there were people about, but eventually I ignored everybody knowing that it was something that had to be done!

Getting through those last couple of days was hard,

really hard at times. I thought I would not make it, all my fears and phobias seemed to surface all at once and I again became preoccupied and withdrawn, spending a lot of time wandering along the beach, not even distracted when I came across pretty girls. I tried desperately to hang on to the thought of the salvation that was just around the corner and tried to subdue the volcano in my head. Gina did not warn me about the effects of the earth and leaves, only asking me to be patient for a little while longer.

The day of salvation arrived and I rang Gina once again and was given instructions to meet her at her shop at noon. I arrived early, half expecting the car to break down or to have an accident on the way, but I arrived safely and waited in a sort of daze for Gina to arrive. As I sat in the car with the sun streaming through the windows I started to feel extremely warm and claustrophobic, and started to panic. I got out of the car and walked up and down the road trying to stay rational knowing I had only minutes to wait. Every person I passed seemed to trigger off my irrational fear about losing control of myself and I had to repeat 'No!' to myself over and over again, clenching my fists in the process. I was so wound up that I did not see Gina arrive and it was not until she called to me that I realised that she was there.

Gina led me into the shop and told me to sit at a table, where she sat opposite me with a bowl in one hand and a book in the other. She put both on the table and I noticed what looked like a couple of black peas in the bowl. Gina noticed my look and explained that the bowl was where the spirit would end up once it had left my body! I was puzzled and told her that I had seen an exorcism before and said that it was nothing like this.

Gina then said that there were many ways of disposing spirits and that this was the way she did it. In reply I said, 'I just want the spirit removed and not destroyed!' She assured me that everything would be all right.

When everything was prepared, Gina then took hold of my hands and uttered what resembled a prayer although she never, as far as I can remember, mentioned the word God by name. She then repeatedly waved her arms, while saying more words. I, meanwhile, felt absolutely nothing, even when she was drawing the spirit out. This was a big disappointment for me as I had been prepared for a rough ride; especially after all I had been through. Gina then asked me to shut my eyes, which I did, and as I sat it went very quiet and all I could sense was a feeling of warmth and a slight hissing noise. On command I opened my eyes and Gina was smiling at me and in the bowl were two black sausage shaped things. I again looked at Gina and she told me that it was all over. The two of us sat and had coffee after the exorcism and Gina asked how I felt. In reply I said it was too soon to say. It was too soon, but I prayed that everything in my life would improve and that I would be a new man. I longed for friendships, relationships and peace. I longed to be able to relax and appreciate the finer things of life, and also I longed to be happy wherever life took me.

As I drove back to Santa Monica I felt a little depressed, but otherwise not too bad. After supper I went down to the Crown and Anchor, where I met up with Chuck who at once told me that, if I wanted, I could work with him in construction after Christmas. With this news I perked up and over a few drinks we discussed the finer details with him. I began to appreciate that Chuck was sticking his neck out for me, especially as he was going to pay cash and I realise only too well the trouble he would be in if the authorities found out!

That night I returned to the construction site and bedded down as usual. I tried to sleep but could not, I started to feel very exposed and vulnerable, and as though I was being watched by someone. I could not stand it any longer, so I rolled up my sleeping bag and put it in the boot of my car and lay in the back of the vehicle and tried to catch some sleep there. I did manage some sleep and when the boss of the site arrived in the morning, I gave him back the keys of the gate, deciding that from then on I would put up with sleeping in the car.

It was the week before Christmas and I was once again working on the pier. The exorcism had made little difference to the way I felt and I was feeling very drained of any real emotions. I had told Gina about that last night on the construction site and she had said that I felt the way I did because I had slept there while possessed, and now I was not, I could pick up the evil residue. Trying to stay calm with this news was not easy because I started to realise that I had been in numerous places while possessed and that was probably why my mental health had not improved. I felt like I was in a nightmare that would not end!

For the first time since I had been in America I started to think about going home to England. I felt the need to be around my family and recognised the need to tackle my problems with my family's help. I did not want to leave Los Angeles, because at last I had the opportunity to earn good wages, perhaps enough to rent my own flat and put down a few roots.

As Christmas was rapidly approaching I contacted the two people who had always made me feel welcome, Sandy and Ray. I told them I was now sleeping in my car so I would return their sleeping bag and I also mentioned my new job, which they were delighted about. They asked me if I had any plans for Christmas and if not would I like to go to their home on Boxing Day? I said I would be delighted, so we arranged it.

On my final day of working on the pier my stress level was very high and I found it hard to celebrate Christmas with my workmates. Presents were exchanged and I received a nice T-shirt from my chosen partner, while I gave her some perfume.

I spent Christmas Day alone, walking round the empty streets of Santa Monica. Every bar and shop was closed but I had taken the precaution of buying beer the previous day, which I drank in my car on the deserted pier while I watched the Pacific Ocean. When I was suitably drunk I fell asleep and thanked God that I was still able to sleep, in spite of everything.

Boxing Day was pleasant, but by then I was depressed so it was hard to enjoy myself. As usual, Sandy and Ray were great hosts and I had plenty to eat and drink. They let me shower, which helped my mood a little and they also allowed me to spend the night on their sofa. By the end of the day I think Sandy and Ray were a little fed up with me thanking them so much!

Depression started to overwhelm me the week after Christmas and I managed to work for Chuck for only two days. It was not particularly hard work but I found it very taxing, and communication with my new colleagues was almost impossible. Chuck was very understanding when I told him that I was returning home due to ill health and I think he realised my predicament was fairly serious.

With my return flight ticket still valid I booked a seat on a flight back to England on the 30th December, which gave me two days to say goodbye to everybody and sell my car. I found a buyer for the car straight away, it was an English lad who wanted it so we arranged that I should hand it over to him at the airport and in return he would give me 50 dollars.

The first people I said goodbye to were Sandy and Ray. It was very hard for me to hold back my emotions as I owed them a lot and wished I was able to stay. I left feeling I had let them down, but I am sure they would have understood my reasons for leaving if they really knew how I felt. Nevertheless, I did owe them a lot and hoped upon hope that some day I would be able to repay them!

On the penultimate night I once again returned to the Crown and Anchor and was pleased to see the Bear was sitting at the bar. We drank some beer together until closing time. Bear got up and shook my hand saying that I would be back. As I settled down for the night in the car I thought about what he had said and wished I had his confidence, knowing that I had to face a battle to keep my sanity and even my life, and to do that I had to go back to England.

My final day in Los Angeles was spent driving to various places, not least to my old spot in the Hollywood Hills overlooking the city. As I stood looking down on it tears came to my eyes as I thought how cruel life could be. I had tried my hardest to get on but circumstances had not been on my side. My dream was over and I must return home to seek a solution and maybe one day find happiness or a least peace of mind.

In the afternoon I visited Gina with a bunch of flowers to thank her for all she had done. She looked a little embarrassed when I gave them to her, but soon recovered to say that I would sleep most of the flight home and would arrive safely. Before I left I told her that if necessary I would ring her from England to seek her advice and she just nodded.

Chuck was in the pub that last evening but he did not stay long. When he left we shook hands and he wished me well, adding that he hoped I would find what I was looking for. I watched him leave and thought again that we could have been great mates. I got drunk for a change and when I left the Crown and Anchor I slipped out the back door not wishing for anymore goodbyes.

The flight left on time, but once again I had to change planes at Houston. Gina was right; I did sleep most of the way back to Gatwick. I arrived on the morning of 31st December getting to Norwich in the afternoon. Mum was expecting me as I had rung her the previous day and we celebrated the New Year together, as a family.

THE SEARCH FOR PEACE

The house in Norwich, which Mum had been buying on my behalf, was not ready yet so I stayed at Mum's house initially. It did not take long to realise that my problems were still with me and were no better since returning from America. I remained convinced that although I was now free from being possessed by the spirit of my Grandmother there was still a lot of its influence still left that affected me greatly. This was particularly so as regards to Mum's house where there were many things that had belonged to my Grandmother still in existence and I knew that I had to get rid of them somehow. There were many things to be aware of although I did not need reminding because I was in a constant state of high anxiety. I had a new purpose in life however, and while I concentrated on scheming and plotting my symptoms seemed under control. My sister, Sue, was also staying with Mum and Tom and she wore a ring, a gold ring with rubies set in it and it was precious to her because it was Nana's old engagement ring, but I had other ideas for it. I bided my time and watched and waited for an opportunity to dispose of it. My chance came one evening when Sue was washing up. Normally she would dry her hands and apply hand cream and immediately put her jewellery back on, but this particular evening she went out of the kitchen to the loo before she had finished. I seized on the opportunity and put the ring in my pocket intending to send it to Gina in America, but before I could do that I had to ride the storm of emotion that erupted when Sue realised the ring was missing.

  At the first possible moment I sent the old ring to America. I did not feel guilty about it because I was convinced it was for the best and I would be thanked for it in the end. By this time I was completely obsessed with removing any trace of my Grandmother from my life and that of my family. Anything, however small and insignificant that I was able to get my hands on was disposed of. Things like crockery and such like were easy pickings as I would pretend to drop them accidentally when washing up. Mum never said anything to me about the disappearances and mishaps, so I assumed she did not realise anything about them and that suited me at least for a while. I even disposed of my Grandmother's gold watch that Mum had given me for my 21st birthday.

My anxiety level was still extremely high and I was getting increasingly withdrawn and retreating into my own little world. Despite all the things I did I could not see any improvement so I rang Gina in Los Angeles as much as I could. Between us we came to the conclusion that whatever I had touched, wherever I had been and whoever I had spoken to in the past, before and while I was possessed, was still affecting me. Gina agreed that she could cleanse my family, but the rest was up to me. Once again, at night, I would pray for strength and beg God to deliver me from the incessant nightmare I was in and beseech him to let no harm come to me and my family.

Realisation grew that until they were cleansed I would have to find alternative digs, because being so close to my family and especially Mum resulted in further anxiety for me. As my house was not ready I was forced to book into the local pub, which was a couple of doors down from Mum and Tom's house. Once again mum did not seem suspicious and seemed to accept the flimsy excuse that I wanted to be independent.

There were so many things to identify and get rid of that I knew it would overwhelm me if I thought about them all at once. I decided to start sorting out my personal possessions when I moved into my new house.

My car, I decided, would have to go immediately. It was a good reliable car that I purchased off Dad before I went to America, but nevertheless, I part exchanged it for a black estate which turned out to be very much less reliable.

My first night in Bed and Breakfast was far from comfortable. I retired after a few drinks in the bar and virtually fell into bed because I was very tired from the usual day's stresses. Expecting a good night's sleep I was very upset when I found that my mind just would not settle, it was as though I was still in bed two doors away. After a while I turned on the light and tried to think rationally as to why I could not sleep. Everything should have been all right because I had never slept in that room before, but something was wrong! As I looked around the room I came across the answer and could not believe my bad luck! The headboard of my bed was identical to the one I used to have on my bed as a child. I did not let it upset me; I just put the mattress on the floor and tried my best to get to sleep there.

The next day I received the go ahead on the house, which was a relief, so I started to move in all my possessions that I had stored at Mum's. I did not have much because I had sold all my furniture, so it was mostly clothes, books and things like that. I quickly bought a new bed which I put in the lounge as I intended to live in one room until I had got myself together. I also arranged for a telephone to be connected as soon as possible so I could have continued support from Gina in America.

There was much to do and the first thing was to rid myself of everything, either sell it or dump it. There were many things that I would rather have kept but I knew that however painful everything had to go! As I sorted through my belongings I was close to tears, there were many things from my childhood like photographs, scrapbooks and certificates that I wanted to keep, so I delayed their destruction hoping somehow that I would be able to hold on to them. I loaded all the saleable things into the car ready to take them to a car boot sale, including my precious leather jacket which I had scarcely had for a year. When I had finished loading I started to put what was left in bin bags ready for dumping. Eventually I came across my prized stamp collection which had been a hobby since I was a young lad and started ripping up every stamp individually. Every stamp, valuable or not, was not spared until I became fed up with this and left the depleted albums for another day. There was also the watercolour painting that Mum and Tom had given me when I moved into my first house. I so wanted to keep it that I rang Gina for advice and she told me that she would bless it for me, so over the phone she said a few words while I repeated them without taking my eyes off the painting. I was thankful that at least my painting was to remain safely with me.

On Sunday I sold practically everything that I took to the car boot sale, mainly because I let everything go so cheaply. My lovely leather jacket was soon snapped up and it broke my heart to let it go.

Any other things that I had left I dumped, all except a few things from my school days, photographs, the watercolour and the remains of my stamp collection which I intended to put up for auction. My house was empty except for those few things and my bed. I still basically felt like shit, so I rang Gina intending to demand answers as to why things were not improving. I did not get very far when I rang because all Gina said was that I had to sell my house because that was also tainted, as I chose it before I went to America and was cleansed!

My life, I decided, was destroyed. I had no friends, I had no job, no possessions and I was soon to become homeless and to cap it all I was still experiencing mental torment! I was still taking Ativan regularly but it seemed to offer little or no support because my stress level was still chronic due to all the distressing thoughts I was still experiencing. All I knew was that I must not give in to the bad thoughts in my mind. I had to stay strong and put my faith in God.

Gina's words stuck with me for the next few days. I tried to make the lounge of the house as comfortable as possible, purchasing a second hand television to watch in the evenings. I did not prepare meals at home at all, preferring to get take-aways or eat out. In fact, I did not use any of the other rooms in the house at all; they all seemed spooky even in the day time! Sleeping was not a real problem although I always had to try and relax my very active mind and thankfully I never seemed to wake up in the middle of the night. However, I still felt uneasy in my house and decided after about a week to book into the Bed and Breakfast further along the road to see if that produced any improvement in my mental state. I still used the house in the daytime to make and receive phone calls and it was not long before I thought I felt a little better which led to me making my mind up that I would sell the house and get a flat or digs for a while until I was better.

The Bed and Breakfast was comfortable, although most evenings I went visiting the local pubs of which there were quite a few. The second day I was there I learnt from Mum that Granddad in Essex was suddenly taken very ill with cancer. Granddad was my last Grandparent still alive and I always considered him my favourite, respecting him a lot, so it was sad to think of him lying in a hospital bed and that night I prayed that he would soon find peace and not suffer too much more.

About four o'clock the next morning, I awoke suddenly and felt a pressure in my chest and a strong feeling of closeness to Granddad. The next thing I felt was anger, because there was no way I would be taken over again, all of a sudden the pressure disappeared. I was stunned and very hurt that Granddad would try such a thing because I admired him so much. Not being able to settle again I decided to get up and ring Gina and tell her the devastating news.

Gina, as usual, took my news in her stride and again offered no sympathy just saying that 'these things happen'. I was getting tired of Gina, she was supposed to be my friend, but never sympathised with me or even offered ways out, I was taking the initiative every time. I decided then that I would stop ringing her and look for other ways to help myself. One thing was for sure that there was no way I would be possessed by another entity; there was no way I would ever let that happen again!

The same week Mum and I went to see Granddad in a hospital in Chelmsford. He was in a lot of pain, had lost a lot of weight and had tubes and pipes coming from nearly every part of his body. We learnt from the nursing staff that they had only just started administering Morphine, which appalled me after seeing what pain he was in. He was still able to speak, however, and told us that he wondered why they still tried to keep him alive, and we were at a loss as to how to answer him. Mum left me alone with him for a little while and that gave me the opportunity to warn him off what I thought he intended, but as I sat next to him I could not bring myself to say anything to him.

That was the last time I saw my Granddad, because he died a couple of days later. With the funeral at the weekend it was a hectic day as the whole family went to pay their last respects. I went reluctantly, because I was still very much on my guard in case I once again had to fend off an invader, but I need not have worried because Granddad never tried to take me over again.

As the opportunities arose I continued my war against my Grandmother's property, although my trips to Mum's died down to once or twice a week. I still felt full of anxiety and my mental health was not improving, but I did my utmost to carry on with life the best I could. I did not change my mind about finding other accommodation and after just a week in Bed and Breakfast I moved into a bed-sit on the north side of Norwich. It was a gloomy place but I felt it would do until things improved.

Decisions at this time, I found, were hard to make with so much going on in my head but, nevertheless, I decided to sell my house. The housing market was booming and had been for sometime, so although I had only owned the property for less than a month I was set to make a healthy profit. I asked my chosen estate agents to advertise it at a cool £7,000 more than what I had paid for it, and did not expect a response so quickly.

Each day, while my house was up for sale, I spent by the telephone in the lounge and passed the time away by watching television (which I took backwards and forwards between my two homes each day). Within a week I had two parties making me offers and actually bidding against each other. I kept ringing each party with news of the others bid and when a price was eventually decided I had made an extra £2,000 over my asking price! I was glad to have sold the house because it meant that I had got rid of another thing from my past, although by now I was getting confused as to why I was not feeling any better. I was still convinced that evil forces were against me and up until then nothing had happened to change my mind.

One evening I was moving my bed out of the house to take to the bed-sit when the telephone rang. I was most surprised to hear it because very few people knew the number and it was due to be disconnected the following morning. Very intrigued, I picked up the receiver. On the other end was a lady who was a friend of Mum's. This friend lived in Somerset and her name was Rita, but by far the most interesting thing about her was that she was a Psychic Medium. By instinct I knew she was going to talk to me about my problems and immediately went on the defensive. However, Rita was a very determined lady and told me that she had looked into me psychically and had found nothing untoward, except the fact that someone was interfering in my life (Gina). We argued on the phone for about ten minutes and by the end I was shell-shocked. Whatever else Rita had done she had planted a seed of doubt in my mind which was to grow very quickly over the next few days. The next morning, when I awoke, there was only what I would call an argument going on inside my head of which I appeared to be a bystander listening to the pros and cons of my meetings with Gina and the subsequent possession by my Grandmother. By the third day, the early morning discussions had more or less abated with my growing realisation that all I had been through the last few months was a lie and everything I had done with Gina in America was one big con on her part. At first I felt such a fool and was ashamed about some of the things I had done, not least stealing my sister's ring and sending it to America.

During the next few days I tried to make up with my family and especially to Sue to whom I promised that I would replace the ring. I described the best I could what had happened, to try and explain my behaviour but the truth was I could not really fathom out the reasons why I had become so involved in the first place.

With the burden of possession over I expected to feel better in myself, but unfortunately this was not the case. My anxiety level was still very high and that in turn seemed to increase my susceptibility for the phobias and fears to be ever present. I found that if I did not concentrate, my thinking would become muddled and confused and I had a big fear that I would become trapped in my thoughts and get sucked in ever deeper so it would be impossible to get out. With these fears always there I tried as much as possible to lead a normal life while still trying to fathom out what was wrong and what was causing it.

Every day was becoming a nightmare, the Ativan I was taking was now having little effect but I continued using it, scared of the consequences if I stopped. The only saving grace at that moment was the fact that I could still manage to sleep pretty well, albeit with the help of a few pints inside of me. I knew that if my sleeping was affected then every problem would become much worse, so I thanked God that I took nothing for granted.

My bed-sit became a little haven because it was a

room at the top of a large house and the rest of the tenants were reasonable quiet, so I was able to shut myself off from the rest of the world when I felt like it which was quite often.

The nearest pub to me was called the Coach and Horses, it was a bit of a dive but most of the locals who used it were friendly, so I was happy there. Pool was very popular there and it was not long before I started to join in, it was the same old story though one game I would play well and the next I would be rubbish, no consistency. Nevertheless, the Coach and Horses became my local and I used it most nights and as time went on my face became accepted as part of the local scene.
The sale of my house went through fairly quickly and a cheque for £27,000 was credited to my bank account. At first I had the idea of wanting to take all the money out and sit and look at it for a while because it did not seem to register in my mind that I was sitting on a lot of money, so there was not any enthusiasm for it. Then, after a couple of days, I decided what to do with it and without any research or advice I bought a 'Financial Times' and picked out five companies that I liked the look of and bought five blocks of shares worth £5,000 each.

Within weeks of buying the shares I started to lose money. The Stock Market, at that time, was in a slump so to have bought shares then was a very risky business. As time progressed the market showed little sign of recovery and by the time 1989 came round I had seen £5,000 of my money disappear. I was not deterred however, and still somehow believed that I was destined to have lots and lots of money. So I continued to take an interest in the Stock Market and as I learnt more about it, it soon became apparent that my money had not been well invested. Although I kept an eye on the market I decided that for a while I would keep the shares I had and hope that things improved.

Dabbling in the Stock Exchange was a stressful thing especially if you lost money, and stress was something I needed to avoid as much as possible. Another worry was what to do with myself because although I had signed on the dole and was receiving a small income I was still dipping into my reserves to fund my nightly trips down the pub. Most days I spent watching television, quite content to watch the world pass me by, but I knew somehow that I would have to lift myself and start making a living again.

Early in 1989 my car was stolen from near the bed-sit. I informed the police and a couple of days later they rang me and said that they had found it. When I collected my car it had been vandalised so badly that it looked beyond repair and this was confirmed a couple of weeks later by the insurance company. This incident made me make up my mind as to what to do. I started looking for a large van with the idea of getting into possibly removals and, or light haulage. When I found one suitable I immediately put an advertisement in the local paper advertising my services.

Optimism was not a quality that I possessed much of, but even so I tried to look on the bright side as much as possible because it was less stressful and without stress I could more or less control the fears and phobias that I had.

While I waited for work to come in I used to be as objective as possible about my problems and without thinking too deeply try to search for an answer as to why I felt like I did.

As the days went by my thoughts once again turned to Ativan and whether it was the cause. I decided not to do anything stupid and rush into a decision, but to register with a local doctor and get his opinion.

As doctors go he seemed quite pleasant, but said that Ativan was fairly safe as regards side effects but could be addictive. He suggested that I try Valium instead for a few weeks to see if my symptoms persisted. I agreed and he started me on a similar dose that I was used to and told me to come back in a month.

It soon became apparent to me that changing medication did not help me in any way, but neither did it make things worse. I stuck with Valium on the doctor's advice for a few months to give it ample time, so I was sure. I had already half planned my next step. When I was prepared, and when I had some spare time I would give up all medication!

Replies to my advertisement had started to come in and for the first few weeks I was busy maybe one or two days a week, mostly with removals. Of course, to make a living I would have to work every day, so I decided to carry on and give it three months. If it had not picked up by then I would have to think again.

Three months came and went and at the end of the period I withdrew the advertisement and started planning my next project. This had been prompted by me meeting a man who knew Mum and Tom and who was currently in business himself. I was desperate to maintain momentum business wise because it definitely helped me if my mind was occupied. I was still far from well however, and no matter what I did to keep occupied I knew things did not improve or even look like improving.

Mum first introduced me to the aforementioned

man (who's name was Arthur) when he told he that he had some work which needed doing and on hearing this, she informed me and we went over to see him. The work involved mixing up different bath salts in machines that Arthur showed me how to use. It was dusty work, but well paid so I was content to do the work hoping that it might lead to other things. While I was there I started to realise how many different combinations of colours and perfumes were possible. These thoughts started to interest me and very soon I had worked out a business plan that I felt sure would be a winner. My idea was to create 12 different types of bath salts and find suitable premises so I could sell them to the public.

    Arthur had no objections to my idea and was only too pleased to sell me the merchandise, so with as much enthusiasm as I could muster I looked for a small shop or unit with which to work from. My search took me to an indoor market in Norwich which seemed quite popular, so being eager to get started I put down a deposit on a vacant unit. I then bought some second hand shelves and other necessary things and set about making the unit as professional as possible.

My small shop opened for business within days, but I soon started to realise that getting the public interested in my bath salts would be a tough job. I found that sitting down all day was boring beyond belief, so I purchased a small teletext television to amuse me through the long drawn out days. With my new toy came the opportunity to keep an update eye on the Stock Market, enabling me to buy and sell shares almost at will.

    It seemed that the only way I could stave off the worse symptoms in my head was to be excited, and the only excitement I could get at that time was to play around with my dwindling capital. Sometimes I would do two or three transactions a day, either buying or selling different shares. I enjoyed being an entrepreneur and often imagined what it would be like if I had millions to play with instead of a few thousand. After the end of every account period (an account period ran normally for two weeks) I received a statement of my dealings from my stockbroker and it was from that that I would know how much I had made or lost.

The shop was a major flop. I stayed with it for a month but it was no good. I received little or no interest from the public. I had spent more or less a £1,000 on the venture most of it going on a new till, which I had stupidly bought. With this loss and the money squandered on the stock market my capital had been reduced to half what it had been when I sold my house six months back. The realisation of this only started to sink in when I was packing up the shop's contents in my van. I began to feel very sick!

After clearing the shop I drove back to my bed-sit feeling very low and empty, knowing that my life was in a mess. It was a warm day and as I became stuck in the traffic something very frightening happened. In an instant a wave of extreme panic came over me, enveloping me in a sheet of emotion, and a very strong feeling of claustrophobia. It was panic on a grand scale and it even surpassed the panic attacks I had experienced in my younger days. For a few seconds I wanted to die, to rid myself of the morbid fear I was experiencing. I reached into my pocket for some Valium, but realised that I had left them at home. I desperately wanted to get out of the van and run, but somehow clung on until the panic started to subside. With relief I wiped my hand across my sweaty brow, put the van into gear and drove slowly the rest of the way home.

It seemed the only friend I had (apart from my family) was time and perhaps drink. After I gave up the shop I tried to concentrate on my problems and somehow wade through my jumbled mind and work out what was the best thing to do. I had to be very careful not to get side-tracked by rogue thoughts however, because otherwise I would waste hours thinking about nothing in particular even though at the time they would seem important.

Eventually I returned to the decision I had made before. I would stop taking Valium or any other drug, but first I would allow myself a little time to see if a regular dose would stabilise my mind. From that day I increased my dose a little and took the medication at set times everyday.

At first, with less stress in my life as well as the regular medication, I seemed to settle down a little, but it soon became apparent that it would be short lived.

Every evening I visited the Coach and Horses and always played pool. My form at the game was as usual up and down, but on the whole I improved with practice. One evening I decided that there were enough people playing regularly to form a second team, so with out much thought about the stress it would put on me I went ahead and formed the Coach and Horses 'B' team. Even though I was trying to stabilise on Valium I made sure that on Thursday evenings everyone turned up to play the pool matches. When matches were away at other pubs everyone used to pile into my van and I would drive them to the venue. One particular Thursday I was not feeling very well, but I still turned out and drove, which meant I could not drink. As the pool match progressed I began to feel claustrophobic, so as a precaution I took another Valium. Within seconds of swallowing it I had the expected panic attack. I ran out side into the fresh air and rode it out, trying to take deep breaths so as to slow down my erratic breathing. When I had recovered I made up my mind to go to the doctor's in the morning because I just could not handle anymore attacks like I have just described.

The following morning, without an appointment, I went to my doctor's surgery and was told there were not any slots for me to fit into so I was forced to wait. While I waited I had another panic attack which was as severe as the previous evenings and apart from gasping for air, I thought I could not swallow either. I leapt out of my seat in desperation and ran up to the receptionist, who seeing my condition immediately called the doctor. I met the doctor halfway down the hall and he guided me into a spare room, after which he tried to calm me down. As the panic slowly subsided, he asked me if I had taken any medication, to which I replied 'yes'. After this he said that the Valium should calm me down instead of the opposite, so maybe I was not taking enough but could not suggest anything else. He told me to increase the amount of Valium I was taking and return the following week.

As I left the doctor's surgery I made another appointment. When I returned to the bed-sit I sat on my bed and contemplated my next move. After a few minutes I came to the conclusion that I had only one choice, and that was to give up taking medication altogether.

After making the big decision to stop taking Valium I became confused and unhappy because, after telling my doctor he referred me to a clinic called The

Bure Clinic, which specialised in treating people coming off drugs, be it legal or illegal. I became unhappy because they told me to come off the medication slowly, over perhaps six months whereas I wanted to give it up completely from day one. I also got a copy of a book called 'Coming off Tranquillisers' which also said where possible slow withdrawal was advisable. The book also listed the symptoms you might expect to experience while withdrawing as well as the benefits of withdrawing. It was a very articulate book and I was impressed except that I decided to reject everything it advised and go 'Cold Turkey'.

THE SEARCH CONTINUES

Within hours of discontinuing the medication my anxiety level hit the roof. I locked myself away in my room for three days and in that time I hardly ate a thing. I drank a lot of tea and smoked numerous cigarettes, and in between these I paced up and down the room. I had read about the symptoms I should expect and recognised that anxiety was definitely one of them. Another worry though was the outside chance of developing epilepsy which, although very slight was very frightening especially as I had developed many of the described side effects mentioned in the book 'Coming off Tranquillisers'.

After a couple of days my anxiety level subsided a little which raised my spirits a bit and gave me hope, but these feelings of optimism were soon dashed by the returning chronic symptoms such as fears and phobias that I had lived with for so long. One thing that did please me was the disappearance of the panic attacks that had plagued me over the last few days.

By the fourth day I was eating properly again and I even went for a drink in the evening, but although I had become drug free in a very short time it was plain to see that all my problems had not disappeared along with them. In fact, as I had a clearer mind the unwanted thoughts seemed more acute than before. My sex drive was as high as ever which meant that my frustration level was also high. I could not remember when my last sexual encounter was and could not see where my next was coming from!

Happiness seemed a world away and I was starting to learn not to even think about the things associated with it. I, at that moment in time, was using all my mental energy in just keeping my mind in check and not let all the unwanted thoughts get out of control. I was still able to appear to others more or less normal except when the slightest trouble threatened, and then I would turn to jelly and lose any remaining confidence in myself. It was not only trouble that intimidated me, it was just the same when a nice girl was around or even a chap I wanted as a friend. These things all made me feel very inadequate!

Life was becoming very arduous and like an assault course, where I had so many obstacles to get over in my mind in any one day. Apart from everything else, I soon started to get a strong feeling that something was very wrong and until I found the answer nothing would change. An obvious statement one might think, but I was constantly, and I mean constantly, looking for an answer in my mind getting into the maze of thoughts and trying to untangle them so I could think clearly and work out what was wrong!

As the summer of 1989 came along I began to get sick of doing nothing and felt that I was still able to do some sort of work. My mind turned to Car Boot Sales yet again, after all I did own a large van which was sitting doing nothing so why not put it to use. I was sitting at home one evening trying to watch television when a brainwave hit me. I was thinking about the way to get stock to sell. I had already tried buying things at auction houses, but found it extremely boring and unproductive so I came up with an idea of advertising for jumble in the local paper and sorting through it. It sounded like hard work for a couple of days a week, but if I planned it right it might be profitable.

As I thought about my new scheme more ideas came into my head. The first thing to do was to rent a garage to store the things and do the sorting in. Once I had a garage I could then advertise, take the calls in the week, collect the jumble on Saturday mornings, sort it out and sell it on Sundays. It sounded straight forward enough, so with no more hesitation I would put my plan into action!

The calls came in thick and fast and I soon started building a stock of saleable items. Most of the things I collected were clothes, so I purchased half a dozen clothes rails and went around the shops scrounging coat hangers and before long it became apparent that I was ready to start trading. There was a large Car Boot Sale just outside Norwich, so I elected to go and try it out and was quietly pleased with the initial results. As the weeks went by I built up a nice business and I remember thinking that it was about time that I started doing something right!

Although I was still managing to do reasonably well, on the inside I was still fighting a losing battle. I thought maybe with the success of my business my mental health would improve, but it did not. By the end of the summer my anxiety had reached crisis level once again. I was still very much aware of everything around me but I was finding it increasingly hard to function properly.

One autumn day at the Car Boot Sale I was sitting on the back of my van, when I started thinking about food and especially chemicals in food. The more I thought about it the more I convinced myself that chemicals in the food I ate were to blame for my present mental state. I had an allergy. Why had I not thought about it before? It seemed so obvious and simple!

When I reached home I comprised a list of all the food that I still thought I could eat, in other words foods that did not contain any chemicals or additives. As the days went by the list grew shorter and shorter, as I seemed to get an immediate reaction after eating things and even produce like eggs and cheese seemed to upset me, which was somewhat of a mystery. Despite many setbacks I continued on the special diet for many weeks although it was debatable whether I felt any better.

Somehow, through adversity, I lived my life as normal as possible although inside I felt far from normal. I still managed to go up the Coach and Horses most nights and I usually drank enough to make me sleep. When I became drunk my world became calmer and I was able to relax more. It was a kind of release for me and in truth it kept me going.

My search for release was relentless, and while I was still on my special diet and sure in myself that much more was wrong and that it was very complicated and extremely hard to find an answer, I once again sought spiritual help.

A lady in Reepham had an advertisement in the local paper offering her services in spiritual matters. I rang her and asked if she did Tarot readings, to which she replied, 'Yes'. So I arranged to meet her the next day hoping to get some answers to the many questions I had prepared. Our meeting was disappointing and frustrating for me, but I did get clarification that there was no curse on me and that there was nothing else untoward happening to me. As for my mental problem, I had got nowhere nearer finding out what was making me feel like I was. However, I did strike up a kind of friendship with the lady whose name was Nikki and promised to keep in touch.

When I was not working (mostly weekends) I had little else to do, so I spent most of the time sitting in the bed sit. I went over to Mum and Tom's twice a week for something to eat, but did not really enjoy doing anything much. Mum tried to please me and took my special diet in her stride, but underneath she worried about me.

When I was with her I used to unload all my worries and concerns on her and she often said that she wished that there was something she could do. It must have been a big strain for her to listen to my incessant talking about the same things day in and day out, but she coped well.

Pamela was a friend of mine. I had met her at a Car Boot Sale and we seemed to get on right from the start. There was not any hanky panky going on between us, for one thing she had a boyfriend, and for another I never looked at her that way, we were just good friends. She lived near me and I was a regular visitor.

She had a dog, a lovely, soppy Alsatian and I loved him and took him out for walks every day! I found him and his mistress very therapeutic for me and I looked forward to my daily visits, which were normally in the afternoons. It was not long before I started doing a few jobs around the house and I even built a fireplace in the lounge, which Pamela was delighted with.

There was another reason why I was a regular visitor to Pamela's. A couple of doors away there was a house that had been repossessed by the Building Society and it needed a lot of work doing to it (just right for me), so I became interested in buying it. Everyday I visited Pamela I would keep an eye on the property that I already considered my own, and eagerly waited for it to be put up for sale so I could snap it up!

With so much turmoil in my life it was a wonder I could make any plans at all, yet alone take on the responsibility of buying a house. If I had looked at my money situation sooner I would have changed my plans a lot quicker than I did, because when I finally worked out what capital I actually had I found that I could not even afford a deposit to buy a house yet alone the monthly repayments on a mortgage. I had less than £5,000 left of my original thousands. I had lost nearly all my money on disastrous share dealings and on ideas for businesses that had fallen by the wayside.

Losing my money was bad news for me, it made my depression worse and cut off another direction which my life could take, it virtually finished any chance I had of returning to the building trade. There were so many negative things happening to me at that time that it started to affect my overall morale which in turn reflected on my mental health making many of the symptoms worse and harder to suppress and control. I started to feel isolated and lonely, and despite my fear of losing control spent as much time with Pamela and my family as I could. I also regularly rang Nikki in Reepham, she had a very calming voice and I always felt better after speaking with her. One day, when I was feeling particularly down I rang Nikki and mentioned to her that I was looking for a good hypnotherapist as I was sure the roots of my problems were to be found in my past. She told me that she knew someone who was supposed to be pretty good, so without hesitation I asked her for his telephone number.

    The hypnotherapist's name was Colin Wilson and when I rang him he said he was sure that he could help me and sounded very confident, so I arranged an appointment with him and felt a little better although impatient for the sessions to start. I was prepared to spend as much money as was needed to find the reason for my problems and at £20 a time it could cost quite a lot of money.

Once again my life was filled with hope and I waited eagerly for my first meeting with Colin Wilson. I had one important engagement before that however. My pool team representing the Coach and Horses had reached the Final of the Area Cup and I was very proud to have led them there. The Sunday night was very special and the event took place at Norwich City Football Club in the Executive Suite. There were other finals taking place as well and there were official referees along with journalists from the local press. I was very nervous and expected to play badly, but somehow when it was my turn to play I concentrated very hard and tried to block every alien thought out of my head and for the duration of the game it worked and I won. With Mum, Tom and Sue looking on my team swept to victory and I proudly held the trophy above my head. The next evening our picture was in the local evening paper and once again I was a proud man.

Colin Wilson was a small man with shoulder length hair and lived in a large house in the centre of Norwich. After greeting me, he showed me upstairs to a room which had two leather chairs facing each other and an untidy desk beside one of them. It was, what he called, his surgery. We started the session with him explaining the sort of therapy he practised. Apparently it was called 'Neuro-Linguistic Programming' and it was achieved under hypnosis. Basically, you would select a period of stress from your past and relive it while under hypnosis then change the way you reacted to it so that it was no longer stressful. He then demonstrated his hypnotic skills and gave me a tape to listen to and said that the next time we met he would do something about my allergy.

Nothing else mattered now. All that mattered was getting well again; it had been so long since I was well that I had forgotten what it was like. I just wanted peace, freedom from the mental torture I had so long endured and a chance to pick up the pieces of my life again, to be genuinely emotional again without interference from alien thoughts. Above everything else I wanted a partner, a lover, someone to share my life with, and someone to be a mother to my children. Somehow I knew though that to have any hope of achieving these things I had more suffering and heartache to go through, but I also knew that Colin Wilson would find the answer to my suffering in one way or another.

Colin did sort out my allergy in the very next session and I was both pleased and impressed. All it took was one period of hypnosis and a few suggestions and I was able to eat whatever I wanted again. After every subsequent session my respect for Colin increased. I became more and more impressed with his positive outlook on life and his undying optimism. I often spoke of him to Pamela and would not have a word said against him and although she tried to talk to me about him I would just shut her out.

There was a lot to do and Colin agreed that if the therapy was to work we would have to be very thorough. He suggested that I make a list of all the adverse things that had happened to me throughout my life so we could tackle everything individually. It would take a long time and a lot of therapy but it would be worth it in the long run. As the weeks went by, I was sometimes visiting Colin two or three times a week and the remaining money I had left was rapidly disappearing. I often felt odd movements in my brain after sessions, which I told Colin about and he said that it was a good sign as the therapy was working.

As we tackled very traumatic times in my life, such as the split up of my parents, I would sometimes have quite violent reactions. These occurred mainly at night and usually consisted of my thoughts becoming very jumbled and out of control, followed by my whole body going stiff and shaking uncontrollably before ending in release and calmness for a short period. I soon began to expect a reaction after every session and was disappointed if none occurred. Colin was pleased when I had a reaction and this served to spur me on and give me further evidence that at last I was on the road to recovery.

As my money supply ran out I started to look at ways to earn more. I was earning roughly £80 a week from my car boot sales, so there was definitely money in jumble and time in the week to expand my operation. I decided on a bold move.

Mum and Tom still had friends in Surrey and kept in contact with them. I knew them as well as they were old neighbours, so I gave them a ring with a proposition. I asked them how they felt about me using their phone number so I could advertise for jumble in Surrey. They seemed pleased to be able to help and said they were willing to list calls as received until I arrived every Monday to do the pick-ups.

So, there it was, at weekends I would work locally around Norwich and on Mondays I would travel down to Surrey and bring a packed van back ready to sort the rest of the week. Within a few weeks I was as busy as I had ever been. It was the summer time so I was doing two, sometimes three Car Boot Sales a week and all the rest of the time was spent either collecting or sorting jumble.

All the money I made went on beer or therapy, so I had little to show for my efforts and it was not long before the pressure built up and I was forced to cease my Surrey operation to reduce my workload.

It was a frustrating time for me because once again I was forced to give up a thriving business as I was not capable of handling the pressure. It was doubly frustrating because while I was under strain I fell out with Pamela in a big way. I was completely to blame because I had become impossible to put up with, for instance, one Monday evening Pamela allowed me to store my entire Surrey jumble in her garage. When I returned on Tuesday evening she had spent all day sorting out the jumble, as she thought that I would appreciate it. In return all I could do was whinge that she had not done it properly and not give her a word of thanks. I also would not hear a word against Colin Wilson which upset her as well. So, what with my constant whingeing and unbalanced behaviour, I lost a very good friend.

Life could not get much worse. Every last hope I had was on the therapy I was having with Colin Wilson. All the spare money I had was spent on therapy and now, after a full year of seeing Colin, it was becoming obvious that my mental health was not improving. I voiced my opinions to Colin, but he said that we should continue with the work for a while longer and try to maintain a positive attitude.

Keeping positive was becoming harder and harder for me. Most of my efforts went towards preoccupation with trying to fight the unwanted thoughts. I was getting no respite from them; from waking up to going to sleep was a mental torture. I used to sit for hours getting entangled with the whirlpool going on inside my brain, getting sucked ever deeper into a maze of thoughts, trying to untangle a ball of string in my mind while remembering to leave a trail to follow on the way out again. I was terrified of getting lost in my thoughts and never be able to get out again, spending the rest of my life floundering in a sea of turmoil and madness. Living a normal life was now virtually impossible, wherever I went or whatever I tried to do I could not break away or separate fantasy from reality. I had to reassure myself that I was functioning in the real world by my sense of touch, sight and smell. That way at least helped me stay in touch with the real world. Drinking was still an escape however, it seemed to dull and slow my overactive mind, although communication with others was becoming more difficult.

People at the pub began to notice my growing isolation and this served to reinforce my solitude. I was past caring by this time, being only concerned with getting my regular alcohol intake! I soon stopped playing pool and communicated less and less with people to such an extent that I sometimes thought that they were all against me and wanted to do me harm. What remained of my hope rested with Colin, I still trusted him and visited him for the therapy as often as I could. I also kept to a rigid routine in my everyday life and lived from day to day, for example: I would do my shopping on the same day every week and another day I would do my laundry and so on.

At least once a week I would go to Mum and Tom's for meal and every visit I would bombard Mum with every aspect of my chronic life. One visit I would tell her I was feeling better, the next I would say I was worse. Whatever I felt, the one nagging thought that never went away was the morbid fear that I would lose control of myself and harm her in some way. Maybe I was brave or just stupid but I still visited Mum regularly.

The next six months were desperate times. I often talked to Colin about work and a career and what I would like to do when I was better, but deep down I knew that given back my money and health I would return to the building trade. I also knew that some things were not possible and I had to be realistic and know my limitations especially at that moment in time. The fact of the matter was I was in no fit state to do any sort of work yet let alone think of a career. Colin persisted and in the end persuaded me to give up my Car Boot Sales and look at the alternative of Market Trading.

One thing I had always enjoyed, whether I was sick or well, was taking money. I was always happy to sell a product for a healthy profit. I found a product that seemed promising and purchased a market stall and went to as many major markets as I could get on. Looking back, I feel that market trading was the only thing I could possibly have done at that time of crisis, and although it was far from easy and my product was seasonal I managed to earn a living for a short period of time and continue therapy with Colin.

As Christmas approached, yet again, my health continued to decline. My anxiety level was sky high and still rising. I was in my own little world and communicated with others only when I had to; all conversation with my family was limited to talking about me and my mental state. My faith in Colin was becoming thin and when I visited him I pushed him more and more for answers. The answers he kept to himself, whilst continuing with relaxation therapy. I still hoped that the money that I was spending on therapy would bare fruit, I also prayed for a miracle.

Christmas was the worst ever, I could not eat because I was too anxious and I was on the telephone to Colin constantly for support. I was desperate and knew I could not go on for much longer. Every thought that entered my head was causing greater and greater anxiety and led onto deeper thoughts that I would hopelessly get lost in. If I really concentrated and pushed all negative thoughts out of my head I could feel like Superman, because the chain of thoughts could work positively as well as negatively. However, once concentration was relaxed negative thoughts soon took over again.

In the New Year (1990), I confined myself to the bed-sit, only venturing out for essentials like food. I still visited Colin and the Coach and Horses but did precious little else. Watching television became an important part of my life, it tended to give my mind something to focus on and I used to very easily become engrossed in whatever programme was on at the time. It helped, a little!

One morning I was watching a programme all about Schizophrenia, and as it went on I started to feel very strange, a sense of recognition and sympathy entered my mind and I felt a sort of numbness in my head which was followed immediately by my hair standing on end. It was really weird and unsettling. I realised that it was too important to ignore and after the programme had finished I turned the television off and pondered over the growing anxiety that I had Schizophrenia. At first I refused to believe it, thinking that it only happened to other people but I did something that confirmed it for me, something that I would not argue with.

The process of praying was not new to me; in fact,

during the last few months it was a regular occurrence. I had mainly prayed for strength and support and it had helped, maybe it was the mere fact of the idea that I was not suffering alone that kept me going. Whatever the reason, I felt my prayers were being answered.

So now that I was being faced with the possibility of having Schizophrenia I needed to be convinced and I knew that if I prayed hard enough I would get an answer. I tried to relax my mind as much as I could and when I felt ready I went down on my knees and asked God to tell me if indeed I did have a psychotic illness.

When I had finished praying I lay on my bed and once again tried to stay as calm as possible. I do not remember how long I lay there, but it must have been a good 10 minutes. Ten minutes does not sound very long, but it was long enough to get an answer and that was all I wanted. To describe how I felt when it came can be put in one word, peaceful. Then came the knowledge that without a shadow of doubt I had been right. Once I was convinced, the peace disappeared and I returned to the turmoil of my tortured mind but the conviction remained, and that was that I did have Schizophrenia!

That very evening I made a few phone calls. Firstly I rang Colin and he told me that he had had his suspicions for some time and would help me all he could. Then I had an emotional talk with Mum, who at first seemed confused and did not want to believe me, but as I talked I became aware of a reluctant acceptance on her part.

Now I knew for certain what was wrong with me I wanted to see a Psychiatrist as quickly as possible. The following morning I went as an emergency to see my doctor. What he told me was not pleasing because he said that it would probably take 4 to 6 weeks to get an appointment at the hospital. I knew my situation was desperate and I could not possibly wait for such a long period, so I decided to try and see a Psychiatrist privately. The same day, without charge, I went to see Colin who I knew had a daughter who was a Psychiatric Nurse. After a session of relaxation, Colin spoke to his daughter on the telephone and came back with the name of a specialist that she had recommended. Armed with this information I returned to my doctor who arranged a private consultation for the following evening.

The next 24 hours were the longest that I had ever spent. I was so anxious that I could not stay still and all I did all day was pace continually up and down my small bed-sit. Every fear and worry troubled me that day and by far the worst was whether the Psychiatrist would believe that I had a problem. To help, I tried to write my symptoms down on paper and hoped that the letter that Colin had said that he would send was also convincing. To cap it all, I then started to worry about the medication I might be prescribed and wondered whether it would work or make me worse!

By the time of the appointment I was a mental wreck and this served to reinforce my story to the man that I pinned all my hopes on. He was Asian, quite small but quite a likeable man and he listened intently to what I had to say. My anxiety was very obvious and I did nothing to cover it up, preferring just to make my problem as believable as possible. The Psychiatrist asked me many questions and was particularly interested in any paranoia I had experienced. At the end of the session he said that he did think I had a big problem, but told me not to worry unduly because there were many anti-psychotic drugs available and they helped a lot of people.

When I was about to leave, the Psychiatrist handed me a letter to give to my doctor and wished me all the best. I handed over £60 and thanked him for his time. I spent another long night without much sleep and thought about how I would feel when I was taking my prescribed medication and how long it would take before it started working. Many fears still plagued me and I once again prayed for strength to see me through the next days and weeks.

My doctor was expecting to see me the next morning and, after reading the letter I had been given, wrote out a prescription. When I left the surgery I read the small, white piece of paper and discovered that I was to take tablets called Sulpuride. I immediately went to the chemists and with the medication that I hoped would save my life returned to my bed-sit. With a little trepidation I took two tablets as directed and then found Sulpuride listed in a book on prescribed drugs that I had obtained from my days of collecting jumble. It confirmed that Sulpuride was an anti-psychotic drug used in the treatment of Schizophrenia.

The next few days I was heartened considerably, because I began to notice a slight improvement in my condition. It was a very emotional time once again, but I tried to stay calm and not over optimistic because I knew too well that life was liable to knock one back!

When the first Friday of being on Sulpuride came along I had been taking it for four days. All seemed well until the evening when I started to get cramp like sensations, first in my teeth and then in my jaw. By the time I was in bed the sensations were becoming very unpleasant and my jaw tended to clamp shut putting a lot of pressure on my teeth. I started to get alarmed, so I rang Colin and told him what was happening. Colin said that it was nothing serious, it was just the medication working through my body and relaxing me.

Eventually I slept, but in the morning after taking more Sulpuride the last evening's symptoms returned with a vengeance. By the time I reached the doctors surgery my mouth was agape and my tongue was hanging out, which was, among other things, embarrassing. My usual doctor was not on duty, so I had to see another who happened to be a woman.

Although I had never met her, the woman doctor seemed to know me and quickly upset me. She started by saying that my immediate problem with my jaw was the side effect from the Sulpuride and would be sorted out by taking Procycladine which was an anti-Parkinson drug. She then went on to say that I should not be on Sulpuride because my problems were emotional and all in the mind. I told her she was wrong and said that she should stick to healing physical symptoms. I felt like saying a lot more because I was very angry, but did not.

When I arrived home once more, I took a Procycladine tablet but as the afternoon approached my jaw problems remained and if anything became worse. Apart from the usual gaping, the reverse sometimes happened where my teeth were clenched and my tongue forced itself back into my throat and choked me.

It was all very disturbing! I once again phoned Colin, but he remained convinced that it was just something that I had to put up with. By this time I was desperate and had no idea what to do, so as a last resort I rang the Yare Clinic, which was a hospital unit for the mentally ill and spoke to a nurse who recommended that I go to the Casualty Unit of the local hospital.

As usual the local hospital was busy, but after I had explain my situation the staff treated me very well and did not keep me waiting too long. After a little while of waiting with my tongue hanging out, the doctor (who had first seen me) returned and explained that I needed an injection of Procycladine as there was not enough in my system to counteract the side-effects of Sulpuride. The drug was administered and within a couple of minutes all the side-effects cleared up and I returned home. Since that time I now take two Procycladine tablets a day and these keep the side-effects at bay.

My overall health continued to improve on Sulpuride and when I had been taking it for two months my condition stabilised and I did not feel too bad, although it did not take me long to realise that I would never be the same as a normal healthy person, but at least I could function at around 80%.

ON REFLECTION

Schizophrenia, even now it is hard to believe, hard to believe that I actually suffer from it. Looking back though and remembering all the suffering and hardship I had gone through, I now do not blame myself and realise it was all down to a chemical imbalance in my brain.

Medication has gone a long way to rectify the imbalance, but a few symptoms persist and those I know I will have to live with for the rest of my life. I have also learnt that stress still plays a big part in my mental health and must be avoided if at all possible.

When I was very young I had very little self confidence and I firmly believe, that as it stubbornly persists even today, that it is connected with the illness. I can say this with confidence because after trying many anti-depressants while seeking further improvement I noticed definite changes in my character (some good, some bad). Since trying the different drugs I have come to the conclusion that, apart from Sulpuride and Procycladine, I am better off without them and as long as I avoid stressful situations I can keep my confidence level up enough to be able to function adequately.

The first real positive symptom of the illness was when I experienced fear while driving on the holiday with Sue, my sister in 1978. I had no idea what was happening to me and really from there started my quest for answers. It was that time when the depression started to creep into my life, which I put down to not having a partner and did not realise the more serious reason.

Many other things happened to help influence me and steer my life down the road it was to take. One example was when on the same holiday I visited the fortune teller on Paignton Pier and what she said came true, thus making me put trust in clairvoyants and spiritualism.

Pressure was beginning to tell on me when I was in my early twenties. I was not a particularly happy man and was very vulnerable even at that advanced age!

Nothing showed off that vulnerability more than when I met Kate. Kate, if you remember was my first love and I went completely over the top with how I felt about her. Looking back, there was no chance of the relationship working because I was too weak and she was an extremely popular and bubbly personality who loved life. The most dominant symptoms of my illness at that time were depression and low self esteem, and whatever I tried to do to alter how I felt simply did not work and in the end I had to learn to live with it.

Around the same time I became friendly with Keith and Linda and consequently learnt about Linda's Mother's gift for reading the future. Due to my lack of confidence and growing depression I needed direction and especially hope in my life, so I felt drawn towards getting a reading done for myself. It's true that when I received a reading I was filled with hope, especially liking the part about the 'Little Lady' with small feet. It seemed somehow connected with Oslo in Norway which was also mentioned, so I grew impatient to meet this wonderful lady thus making up my mind to go to Oslo! As you have already read, my trip proved fruitless except to prove the reading right and give me hope that the rest would also come true!

Thus began my search for happiness and my belief that my destiny lay possibly abroad in some foreign country. When I left for France I was, once again, full of hope and excitement. As it turned out the trip was full of adventure and I enjoyed most of it. In hindsight I now feel I missed some opportunities through the lack of confidence and my preoccupation with trying to find 'my dream lady'. I now know that relationships play a very important part in shaping our lives and at that stage in my life when I was not too ill I had chances to form relationships with the opposite sex but sadly, through various reasons 'missed the boat'.

Throughout my trip to France I did get hints of the illness, not least as I have already described on the station at Avignon, when I was drawn to jumping in front of trains! I never did it, however, but the experience did upset me and must have added depth to subsequent bouts of depression and confusion.

My next trip abroad had its moments and again I was presented with opportunities to get off with the opposite sex. My first chance came when we were grape picking in Bordeaux. To refresh your memory, she was the one who I found sitting on my bunk when I returned late from the dining room. We had previously been talking about sex and it was patently obvious what she wanted, obvious that is to everyone except me. I do not know what she thought when I did not take the bait but when it finally sank into my head I once again hated myself and became even more frustrated. Even from an early age I have had a blockage (for want of a better word) in my thinking where I find it hard to think that any female would actually fancy me!

As I continued my trip and started hitch hiking I can honestly say that I enjoyed every minute. I loved the variety and the uncertainty every day threw at me it gave me little time to be depressed and consequently less time to think about myself. I even felt more confident for a time. However, when I stopped travelling as I reached Copenhagen, depression soon returned abruptly. Even my decision to make the journey to Copenhagen was suspect. I still had the obsession that I was going to meet my 'Little Lady' and felt my destiny was in Scandinavia. I was clearly suffering from the onset of the illness.

When I returned from Europe I had my first mini breakdown which disturbed me greatly, and immediately after that I was put on Ativan for the first time. To complicate things, around the same time the unwanted negative fears started to affect me (probably triggered by the breakdown); I had suffered with them before but not so prolifically. I was getting very confused by events, not knowing what was going on and still under the illusion that everything would eventually be all right.

The only positive help I had, looking back was the Ativan, but even then I fought against taking it regularly. The absurdity of the illness was that it could so easily be mistaken as a nervous complaint and to the outsider that is what it must have seemed. It certainly fooled me although I should have paid more attention to the psychotic thoughts I was having and even the depression, which was a big problem.

All through my adult life I had liked a drink and as long as I did not over do it, it had always been therapeutic for me. In fact I feel that drink played a very important part in my life, making me relax and forget my troubles for a couple of hours a day, and without it I feel the illness would have destroyed me.

Spiritualism played a very significant part in my life. As I was always looking for answers to my problems I was particularly vulnerable to this sort of religion and the practices therein. The evening that I witnessed the exorcism proved to have a big impact on the direction my life would take. The moment the seed of suspicion was sewn in my mind I always veered towards thinking that I was somehow being influenced by evil. This theory was especially brought into importance when I visited America, the results of which you have already read about and will be reflected upon later in this chapter.

Another thing that I experienced was the strange silent telephone calls. I still believe that they were somehow connected to the Spirit World. At the time they occurred I was not very well at all and I tended not to think about them very hard, but now after the event I can see no other explanation but remain confused over their significance. Even now I would like to believe that I have a soul-mate waiting for me in the afterlife and somehow link her with the telephone calls, but it is all conjecture and I shall take the mystery to my grave. I remained convinced that the calls were to help me in some way and were nothing but good and when I wanted them to stop they did.

My search for peace and a life took me to Los Angeles and even more problems. It was not my initial intention to go and see a psychic, but as the pressure built up I started, once again, looking for answers. The first person I saw told me what I wanted to hear (I was cursed) and, of course, when I finally saw Gina I was putty in her hands.

My first encounter with Gina was when she told me I was possessed by the spirit of my Grandmother, maybe I had let it slip out in the conversation without realising it but one thing was for sure she received no argument from me and right from the start I believed it. Now, of course, I know Gina was conning me, but at the time I was so sure that she was a good, honest person who genuinely wanted to help me. I am sure the illness played a big part in influencing my judgement and made me more vulnerable, because even when Gina said that she was working hard at night for me, without me feeling any better, I still believed her bullshit!

The truth about Gina is that she is a nasty, evil

woman who preys on weak and vulnerable people and cons them into handing out large amounts of money. She is doubly evil because she has been given a talent or gift, if you like, but she uses it to promote wickedness by which she lines her own pockets.

Los Angeles was, without a doubt, a violent city and I witnessed various events to prove this, but in spite of it all I met some really nice people. I came to know Chuck quite well after meeting him in the Crown and Anchor, he got me the job working on the pier and he also risked his own job by employing me in the construction trade. Chuck and I could have been very close mates had things been different. Towards the end of my stay in America I think he realised something was wrong with me and when I left he wished me all the best. Sandy and Ray did so much for me it was untrue.

Without their help and especially Sandy's support I would have been in a lot of trouble. I still think about them today and wish that I had left on better terms, but unfortunately events did not allow it. I owe them a lot and feel sure that one day, maybe not in this lifetime but one wonderful day I shall meet with them again and repay their generosity and rekindle our friendship.

Once back home in England I still believed that I was being influenced by something sinister. I still looked to Gina for support and ran up quite an expensive phone bill. The truth was that by this time my illness was becoming chronic and it helped to concentrate or preoccupy my mind with something, rather than get lost in the turmoil of thoughts that plagued me. Once I no longer thought that there was an evil influence on me it was not long before another obsession took over, namely thinking I had a bad allergy, and so it went on.

Even when I gave up taking Ativan and Valium I

suffered all the side effects in the book I had read.

Towards the end I believed every thought that was predominant in my mind. Once again, I concentrated my mind and put all my trust in another person, a person that would ultimately take more than £3,000 off me in the name of therapy, his name was Colin Wilson!

Every ounce of trust I had, I gave to Colin. I had to fully commit myself to him to believe in him for my own welfare. Once again, looking back, the many months I spent with Colin were a complete waste of time and money. To make matters worse, after certain sessions of so called therapy, I experienced what I thought to be reactions to it when really all it was all the time was the illness. Apart from the obvious thought disruption, the illness often upset me physically and sometimes I felt pressure and movement inside my head.

Colin Wilson must have known what was wrong with me long before I did, but continued to take my money and worst of all, allow my suffering to continue longer than it should have done. At the end, when I saw the Psychiatrist I was virtually at the end of my tether. I feel sure that I could not have gone on much longer with what I now describe as 'The Mental Torture' I was going through.

My family, especially my Mum, put up with a lot while I was ill. The possessions of my Grandmother that I tried to destroy, and in some cases succeeded were understandably of sentimental value to Mum but she took it in her stride and was more worried about my welfare. As in most cases of mental illness, people close to the sufferer are affected and I am just thankful that during times of crises I had a family that stuck by me. Unfortunately, and maybe understandably, friends are not so tolerant. I lost some good friends while I was ill, including Pamela who was my first real friend on my return to Norwich.

Finally in this chapter I want to mention my dear old Grandfather who died when I returned from America. I never had a chance to pay my last respects to a man who I looked up to and admired. Even when I visited him in hospital I was too involved with my own problems to say goodbye and even thought that he wanted to invade my own body which, of course, was ridiculous. I hope that he now knows what I truly felt and still feel about him and the fond memories I have of him. God bless him.

HOW IT IS NOW

Well, it has been over five years now since the

confirmation that I had a psychotic illness and I am coping pretty well. I shall never be 100%, but the medication I am on keeps me at around 80%. I have my good and bad days and I have learnt to expect no further improvement. As well as coping with the illness I have come to terms with the adverse effects of taking medication. The first thing to occur was significant weight gain. I put on an extra five stone in the first six months and now remain in excess of 17 stone. Apart from the weight gain there are a few more minor adverse side effects due to the medication which include tiredness and lowering of the sex drive.

About a year after diagnosis I moved from the bed-sit and with the council's help obtained a rented flat, which I am very happy with. Although I do not work and I am very unlikely to ever again I receive adequate benefits with which to live on. I still visit the pub when I can afford it and have the luxury of having a number of drinking houses in my vicinity of which to choose from. Drinking remains a very important part of my life as I still use it as a means of escape.

As a result of the illness I have become very involved with matters concerned with mental health and go to various meetings in the mental health field. Apart from giving me something to do, I enjoy debating and have a genuine interest in trying to improve the life of people with serious mental problems. In my spare time I am lucky to be able to enjoy watching television and lose myself in a programme and not think about my life, as that would be unproductive and stressful.

My relationship with my family is now very good. Mum accepts that I am mentally ill and supports me all she can. I still visit at least once a week (usually on Sundays) and I enjoy her company to a point that I sometimes feel guilty that I do not see her more often, because she is not getting any younger and our time together is precious to me. Maybe if I did visit Mum more I would start taking her for granted, which is the last thing that I want to do. Also, sometimes my emotions are all 'screwed up' so I can not always rely on them to be genuine. One thing I do know is that Mum is my favourite person in the world and I know that I love her although I never tell her, and I do not know what I would do without her.

Tom is a very generous man and very self-opinionated. He never mentions my illness but there again nor do I to him, but I am sure he is aware of my problems and supports Mum where he can, as they are very close. Since Tom has retired he is much more relaxed and approachable and although he sometimes has his moods I find that I have a lot more time for him than I used to have. I have known Tom for nearly 30 years now and he has been there to support 'us children' when our real father has not, so I know that if anything ever happened to him I would miss him a lot.

My sister, Sue, is now living with a man called Kevin and she seems happy enough, which I am pleased about. I think she mostly understands me, but maybe sometimes forgets my limitations. However, that aside, she often invites me over for meals and things and comes to Norwich for a drink so I see her quite regularly. We are close and I would not swap her for anyone else that is for sure.

She is closer to Dad than I am although neither of us sees him that often. I have never been with Dad long enough, all through my life, to really get close to him but I do enjoy being around him when Hazel's not about. He lives in Spain most of the year, only coming back to

England for three months in the summer. When he is in England he lives in a mobile home on the Essex coast and visits us maybe three or four times during his stay. I have visited him occasionally but it is always soured by the presence of Hazel. I will always regret not spending more time with Dad, but looking at it in reality there has always been obstacles in the way. First of all, Dad has always been a little selfish and puts his own interests first which is very annoying and trends to put you off staying with him, but by far the biggest obstacle is Hazel.

My illness means nothing to Hazel; in fact, she tends to believe that there is nothing wrong with me. I refuse to let it get me down and for the little time I see her I plat along with her and act as though she is right, behaving like a fat, lazy, good for nothing like she thinks I am. I think enough has been said except that because of Hazel's behaviour I have been restricted in how close I have been able to get to my father and that I will never forgive or forget!

Since I have been on medication I have had to come to terms with certain things in my life. Throughout my late teens and twenties I used to dream of meeting some special person and settling down and maybe having a couple of children. Now I have had to face reality and train my mind not to dwell on such things or I should surely cause myself undue stress which could lead to serious complications. Eventually after making a conscious effort to restrict my thoughts I have found that I do not think about the subject anymore. It is sad, in a way, to restrict your dreams but I have had to face reality as I said and keep my stress levels down.

Occasionally, usually after I have had a drink, I get

sentimental and play a few soppy songs and think about love but come the morning it is all forgotten about. I now take joy in seeing young, happy couples together and wish them every happiness for their future. I also take joy in seeing people pair off because I still believe that, apart from people with *serious* mental health problems, everyone has a potential partner waiting for them somewhere and I hate meeting lonely people.
One day I know I will be happy and this is due to my beliefs in an afterlife and reincarnation (which I will write about later on). I honestly and truly believe there is someone very special for me, but when and where I shall meet her I do not know except to say that I do not expect to meet her in this life.

    Sometimes, as I have said, I do get sentimental and it is then that I feel sorry for myself knowing that I have not even kissed a girl for six years, yet alone slept with anyone. Although the medication has affected my sex drive it has not completely, so sometimes I do still get frustrated and long for a quick fling with some willing female! If there is such a thing as reincarnation, next time round I hope I will be able to chat up girls because in this life the illness inhibits me to such an extent that I have not got a chance, so now I do not even bother!

    One thing that I have experienced in this life is love, or at least the feeling of being in love. As memories fade with time the one girl that remains in my thoughts is the one I knew least about. I have mentioned her briefly earlier in this book. She was the girl who was the barmaid in my local pub (the Hen and Chickens in Bisley), who was married at that time. I met her about a year later after I had moved to Bagshot and found out that her marriage had failed, and then as we grew closer I made a right fool of myself one fateful evening and lost her for good. I now do not blame myself for that mistake because I was ill and under a lot of stress. Out of the few girls I have loved she remains the dearest and I can not even remember her name!

Life on benefits is comfortable but boring. I sometimes wish for my building days to return, but I realise that it is now no longer possible. Even if I was mentally fit to work I could not return to building because my back is not strong enough. If I had continued building, and especially renovating and improving properties, I would have been a wealthy man by now. Occasionally, especially after a drink, I allow myself the pleasure of dreaming about how my life would be without mental illness. I would have a nice big house with a couple of cars, a very healthy business with employees, lots of business associates and friends, but most importantly a beautiful wife and at least a couple of children!

Instead of living, I exist from day to day watching each wasted day go by. I try to be constructive by involving myself in the improvement of mental health services, but I am afraid it is no substitute for a healthy brain. I would like to think that God had some purpose for me leading an unproductive life, one day I might find that I have achieved something maybe by improving the lot of my fellow sufferers. I hope so, I would love to improve the life of my peers because they suffer enough and often in silence.

One thing I believe, above everything else and has kept me going, especially during the last few years, is my belief that there is a God. I do not pray a lot, I feel I do not need to because I am sure he knows my thoughts and intentions as well as I do. Do not get me wrong, I still believe in the power of prayer and do pray sometimes, but I still believe that God knows what sort of person I am and I often speak to him either in my mind or occasionally out loud. You would expect that as I am mentally ill and have had my life ruined by my illness that I would have little time for or faith in God, but that is not so because I believe that I have and am still suffering for a reason and that when I die I will know that reason and have it justified.

Although I do not look forward to the process of dying and pray that it will be quick, I do look forward to being free of this earthly body so that I can be like everybody else and have a healthy mind or soul or whatever you want to call it. You must have gathered by now that I believe in the afterlife and do not believe that when people die that is the end of existence.

Life to me is all about experiencing and going through everything it throws at you, learning as you go, so that you are (when the time comes), a better 'being' for it. I do not now why I have had to suffer in this life, maybe I chose to or maybe it is some sort of punishment for being 'naughty' in another life, which brings me back to the subject of reincarnation.

I would love to have another chance of living, but next time with a healthy brain. I possess a few books which discuss the subject of reincarnation and faced with certain evidence, i.e.: Past Life Regression, I have come to believe that you just do not live once. This is of some comfort to me especially when I feel bad. When that happens I dream of being in another body and living as an equal to everyone else, but still being me with my own unique personality. I dream that I would be popular and well respected, and be successful, but most of all happy!

Coming to terms with being mentally ill has been

hard, but necessary. I have had to accept that I can not do certain things that healthy people take for granted. I have already mentioned the negative effect I have on women but I have not said how it has a knock on effect in respect to enjoying other things. I do not go to night clubs anymore because I see so many attractive women that it just makes me frustrated. The same happens when I am walking in the crowded centre of Norwich, by the time I return home I am so miserable it takes an hour to recover, especially in the summer. I have not had a holiday since my last, disastrous, trip to Spain almost ten years ago. Now I am receiving generous benefits I could afford to go but I remain in two minds whether to spend so much money on what could prove to be equally frustrating!

When I am at meetings I am usually with men and very few women, so I stay reasonably stable and that remains so when I am at home. When watching television I tend to be very moved when something sad happens or when there is a happy reunion or such like. Sometimes through the haze of medication I sit and imagine that one morning I will wake up from the long nightmare of mental illness and I will be normal and healthy with ambitions and dreams once more.

Occasionally I think about how much mental illness has changed my life. It is like walking down a country lane and reaching a fork in the road, where the left-hand one is bright and sunny and lined with a beautiful avenue of trees covered in cherry blossom but it has a padlocked gate barring the way. Meanwhile, the right-hand lane is dull and gloomy with storm clouds overhead and no leaves on the trees. This one has no gate and is accessible so you have to take it. You wish you could take the other one but the gate is too high to climb.

Some days, for example on a lovely spring day after a long winter when glimpses of emotion filter through the haze in my mind, I sometimes think of that elusive left-hand fork in the road and long for another chance at life but I know that this can not be this time around, but maybe in the next life I can be the real me!

THE END!

A Can of Madness

By Jason Pegler

Britain's answer to Prozac Nation is the book that inspired the setting up of Chipmunkapublishing. This autobiography on manic depression takes you to the edge of the abyss and then helps you to recover.

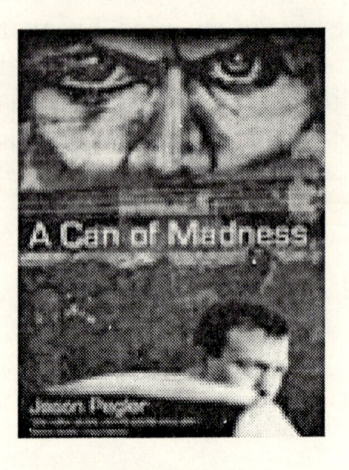

Order online or write a cheque made payable to Chipmunkapublishing for £12 and send it to Chipmunkapublishing, PO Box 6872, Brentwood, Essex, CM13 1ZT.

ISBN 09542218 2 6

WWW.CHIPMUNKAPUBLISHING.COM

World Is Full Of Laughter

By Dolly Sen

The acclaimed autobiography on manic depression and child abuse.

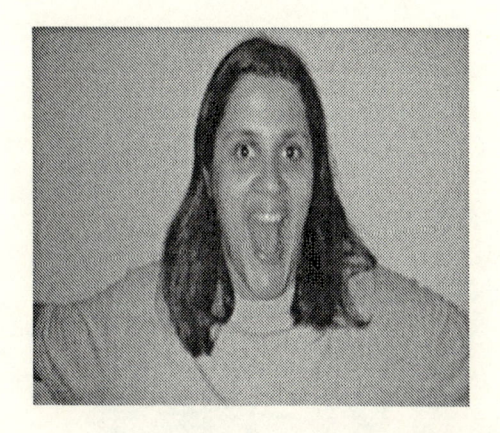

Order online or write a cheque made payable to Chipmunkapublishing for £12 and send it to Chipmunkapublishing, PO Box 6872, Brentwood, Essex, CM13 1ZT.

ISBN 0 9542218 1 8

WWW.CHIPMUNKAPUBLISHING.COM

The Naked Bird Watcher

By Suzy Johnston

The highly acclaimed and positive autobiography on manic depression from a talented lady in Scotland.

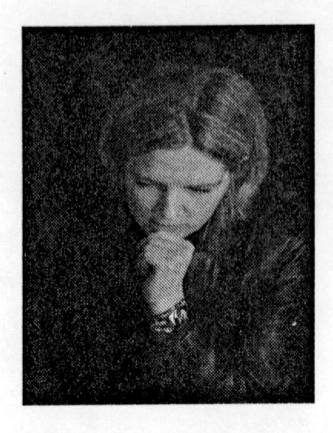

Order online or write a cheque made payable to Chipmunkapublishing for £12 and send it to Chipmunkapublishing, PO Box 6872, Brentwood, Essex, CM13 1ZT.

ISBN 0 9542218 3 4

WWW.CHIPMUNKAPUBLISHING.COM

Who Cares?

By Jean Taylor

An autobiography on manic depression from a survivor and carer from Blackpool.

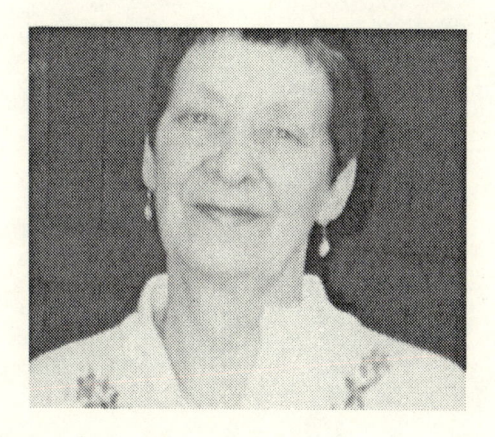

Order online or write a cheque made payable to Chipmunkapublishing for £12 and send it to Chipmunkapublishing, PO Box 6872, Brentwood, Essex, CM13 1ZT.

ISBN 0 9542218 5 0

WWW.CHIPMUNKAPUBLISHING.COM

The Necessity of Madness

By John Breeding

A counselor and activist tells us in a simple way how madness is a metaphor and psychiatry is a clinical construct.

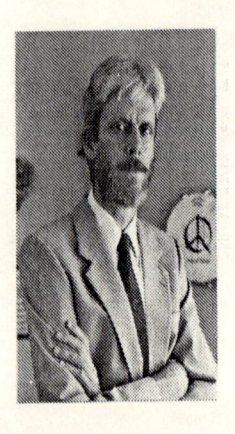

Order online or write a cheque made payable to Chipmunkapublishing for **£30** and send it to Chipmunkapublishing, PO Box 6872, Brentwood, Essex, CM13 1ZT.

ISBN 0 9542218 77

WWW.CHIPMUNKAPUBLISHING.COM

Poems of Survival

By Sue Holt

Powerful poetry of a manic depressive battling for survival. Extremely moving and honest.

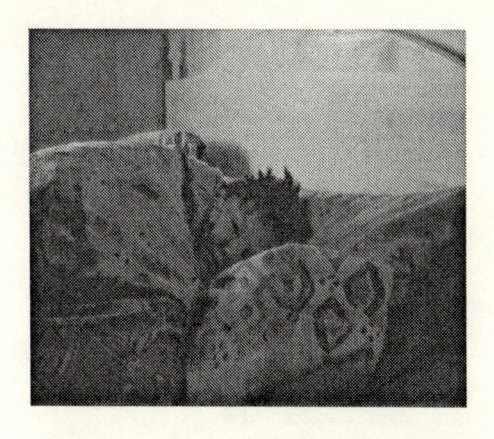

Order online or write a cheque made payable to Chipmunkapublishing for £12 and send it to Chipmunkapublishing, PO Box 6872, Brentwood, Essex, CM13 1ZT.

ISBN 09542218 9 3

WWW.CHIPMUNKAPUBLISHING.COM

Don't Look Back In Anger

By Phillip Pettican

An autobiography on Schizophrenia with an amazing transformation half way through the book.

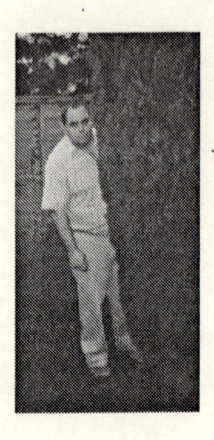

Order online or write a cheque made payable to Chipmunkapublishing for £12 and send it to Chipmunkapublishing, PO Box 6872, Brentwood, Essex, CM13 1ZT.

ISBN 09542218 6 9

WWW.CHIPMUNKAPUBLISHING.COM

Love Is A Spider's Web

By Queen Irena

This sensuous mother of seven and care has a real story of survival to tell.

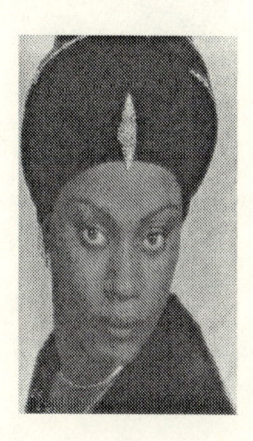

Order online or write a cheque made payable to Chipmunkapublishing for £12 and send it to Chipmunkapublishing, PO Box 6872, Brentwood, Essex, CM13 1ZT.

ISBN 19046970 0 3

WWW.CHIPMUNKAPUBLISHING.COM

Why Me?

Tony Hurley

Experiences of manic depression from an open university graduate.

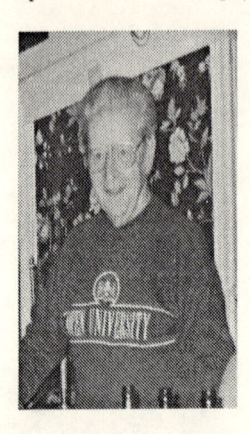

Order online or write a cheque made payable to Chipmunkapublishing for £12 and send it to Chipmunkapublishing, PO Box 6872, Brentwood, Essex, CM13 1ZT.

ISBN 190469702 X

WWW.CHIPMUNKAPUBLISHING.COM

A Can of Madness Play

Adapted for stage by Robert Hutchinson and Jason Pegler

Sit and understand manic depression for the very first time, you can see how manic depression feels from the inside

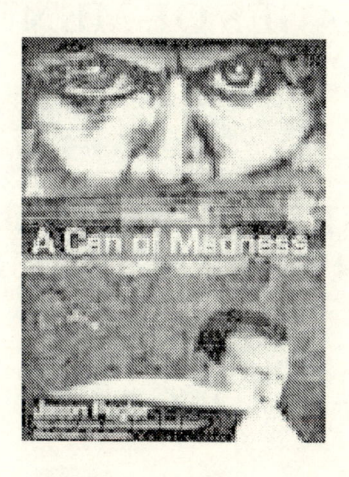

ISBN 1 9046970 1 1

WWW.CHIPMUNKAPUBLISHING.COM

First showing February 2003

Chipmunkapublishing

PROMOTING POSITIVE IMAGES OF MENTAL DISTRESS

THE MENTAL HEALTH SURVIVOR'S PUBLISHER

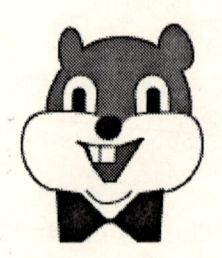

WWW.CHIPMUNKAPUBLISHING.COM

Printed in the United Kingdom
by Lightning Source UK Ltd.
9744200001B/2